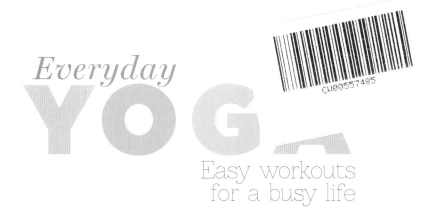

Everyday YOGA

Easy workouts for a busy life

Words and yoga instruction Eve Boggenpoel
Editor Mary Comber
Art editor Kelly Flood

Photography Kirsty Owen and Danny Bird @ Tapestry
Hair & make-up Nathalie Fournier and Danielle Hudson @ Artistic Licence
Models Halla Kopel, Emily Eaton and Kim Hartwell @ WModel

Publisher Steven O'Hara
Publishing Director Dan Savage
Marketing Manager Charlotte Park
Commercial Director Nigel Hole

Printed by William Gibbons and Sons, Wolverhampton

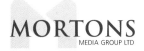

Published by Mortons Media Group Ltd,
Media Centre, Morton Way,
Horncastle, LN9 6JR
01507 529529

CONTENTS

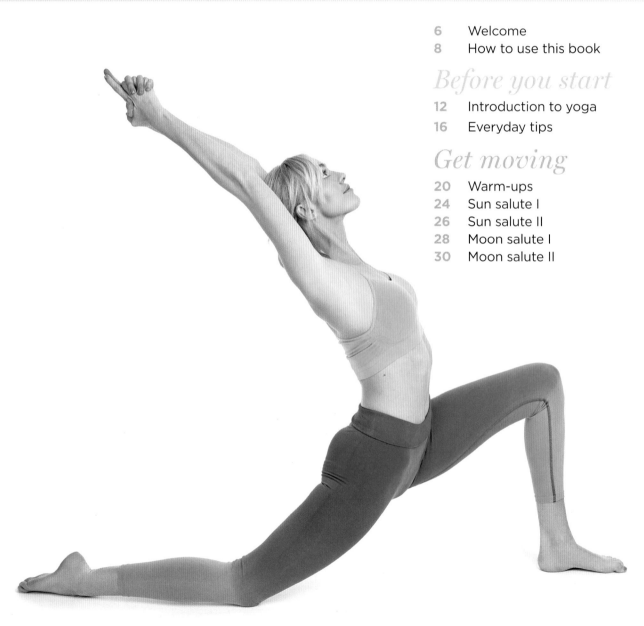

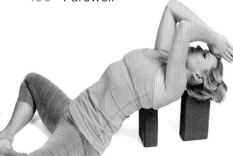

WELCOME!

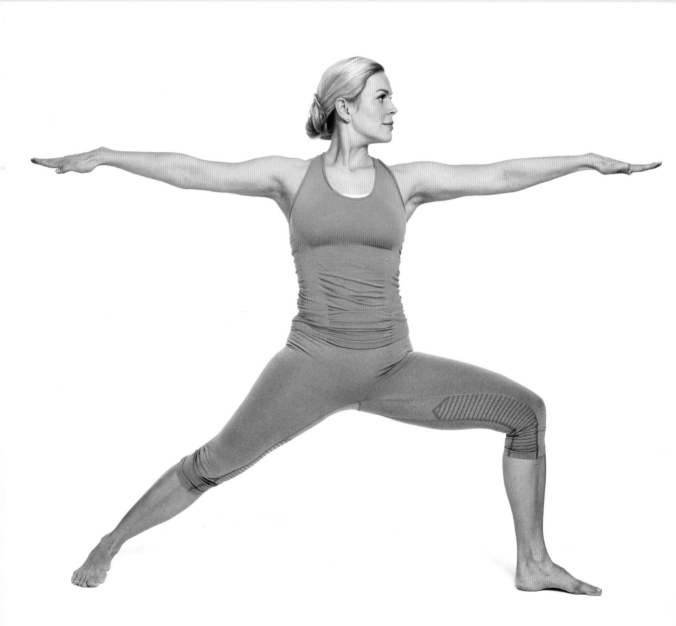

_Yoga is a beautiful way to bring calm
and presence into your life, but it can do far more_

This ancient practice not only helps ease stress, it can also refresh you after a poor night's sleep, boost your energy and heart health, help you get back on form after an illness, increase your fitness for other sports or speed up your recovery after injury. Yoga increases confidence, sharpens concentration and makes you feel more centred and grounded.

As with most activities, the more you practise, the better the results which is why we've written _Everyday Yoga_. In this book, we've chosen five yoga styles — Iyengar, Sivananda, Vinyasa, Yin and Restorative — each with one or two sequences you can practise on a daily basis. That way you can tailor your sessions to help you achieve your goals, whether it's to build your strength for another sport, banish insomnia, beat back pain or bring more mindfulness into a hectic work and family life.

I hope that as you learn more about the different qualities these styles can bring to your practice, you find one (or more) you can turn to day after day to give yourself the love and attention you deserve, every day, to help you live the life you were born for.

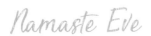

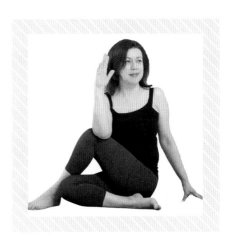

ABOUT THE AUTHOR

Eve Boggenpoel has been practising yoga and meditation for 25 years. Self-taught initially, her formal yoga journey began with a German Iyengar teacher when she learnt to value the significance of good alignment. She went on to include Vinyasa and Yin styles with inspirational teachers Shiva Rea, Sarah Powers and Simon Low.

Eve is a qualified homeopath and health journalist, and author of several MagBooks, including _Yoga Calm, 10-Minute Mindfulness, Yoga Cures_ and _Yoga, A Beginner's Guide._

7

HOW TO USE

Can't wait to get started? Read these guidelines first to make sure you get the most out of your practice

A slower heart rate, a calmer mind, more focused energy... just 10 minutes of yoga can make a significant difference to your day. And this book offers a series of postures and sequences in five different yoga styles to help you achieve just that – and more. It will also help you relax deeply, build strength and find more purpose in your life.

If you work with the postures on a regular basis, even the more challenging poses will become more familiar to you and you'll start to relax into them, understanding your body and its limitations, as well as fine-tuning your alignment. To stay safe and injury free, work through the book in sequential order. Once you have more experience in the different styles, you can either hone in on one that works for you or mix and match your sessions according to your needs on the day.

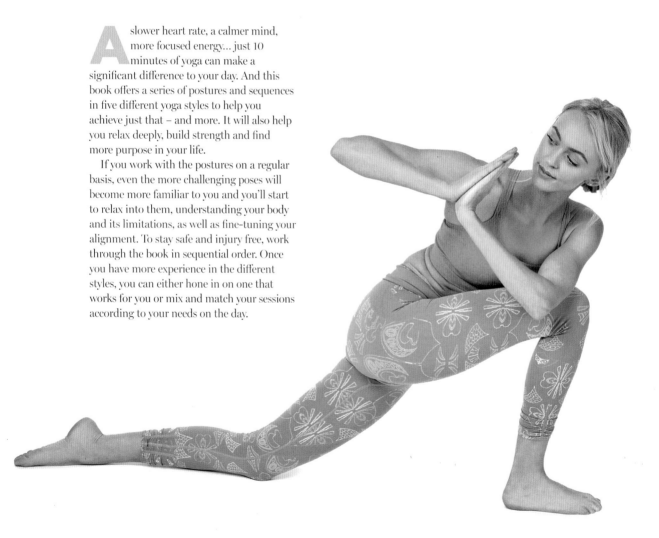

this book

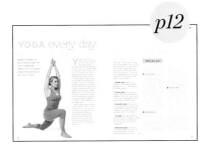

p12

1 INTRODUCTION

Find out how to make a daily yoga session part of your life, and discover how to tailor your sessions to match your goals using the five styles of yoga in this book.

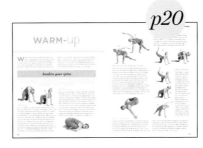

p20

2 WARM YOUR BODY

Prepare your body to practise, and prevent injury with moves that warm up your spine, open your hips and free your shoulders.

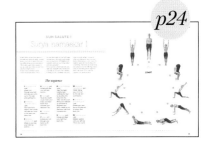

p24

3 START MOVING

Now that you're feeling more fluid, chose one of four Sun and Moon salutes to suit your needs on the day. Choose from calm and gentle, to strong and energetic.

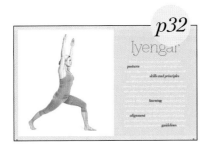

p32

4 DISCOVER YOUR YOGA STYLE

Read about the yoga style you've chosen and how it can help you meet your goals. Learn a meditation and a pranayama technique to deepen your practice.

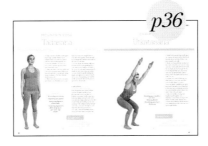

p36

5 THE POSES

Here you'll find in-depth guides for getting into the postures safely, learn their individual benefits and find tips to help you practise them with ease.

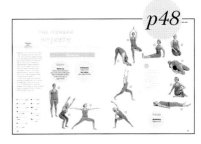

p48

6 THE SEQUENCES

Once you've learnt the poses, it's time to put them together in a daily practice. Whether you have 10 minutes or an hour for your session, there's a sequence to help.

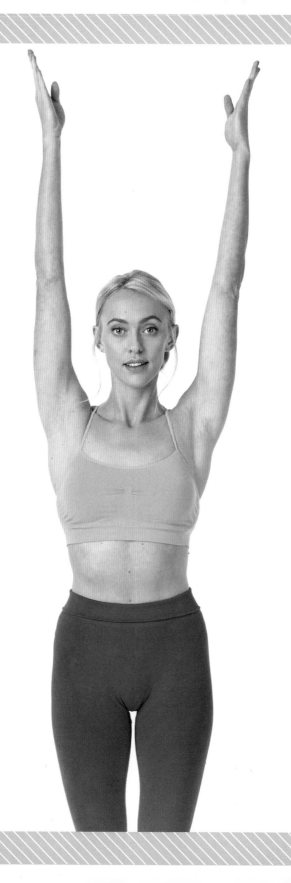

Before you start

Ready to begin? *In this chapter we'll show you how you can create a regular home practice in your life – no matter how busy you are! You'll learn the* **benefits** *of doing yoga every day, discover how it can change your fitness levels, boost your health,* **banish stress** *and improve your overall* **wellbeing***. You'll find out how to tailor your practice to suit your specific needs, so that instead of joining a general yoga class where one size has to fit all, you can make yoga work for you, whatever is happening in your life. You'll learn about the* **five different yoga styles** *in this book so you'll know which to practise and when, and discover 21 ways to help you stay on track with your sessions, to make sure you enjoy the benefits of yoga* **every day** *of your life!*

YOGA *every day*

Want to shape up,
ease stress, improve
your wellbeing?
Here's how to create
a tailored practice to
suit your needs

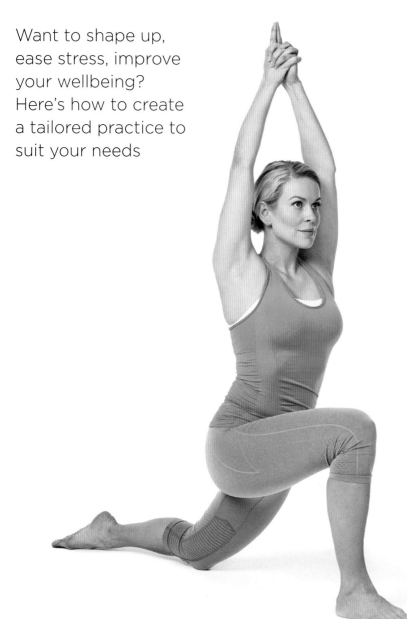

Yoga has never been more
popular. Studios are popping
up in the smallest of towns
and on the top floors of city
skyscrapers, new classes are available on
your smart phone, on your office rooftop
or with a private teacher leading group
sessions in your front room. And it's not
surprising, more and more people are
enjoying its transformative powers.

Practising yoga on a daily basis has
myriad benefits. On a physical level, it
strengthens your muscles, protecting
your joints from strain; it boosts spinal
health and builds bone strength; it thins
your blood, reducing your risk of heart
attack; it boosts immunity; it reduces
high blood pressure; it lowers excessive
cortisol and blood sugar levels; and it
increases your heart rate and helps you
lose weight. If yoga was available as
a pill, doctors would be handing it out
on a regular basis!

But the benefits of yoga go further,
a regular practice increases your focus,
calms your nervous system and has
been shown to beat depression and
promote feelings of happiness by
increasing the production of the
neurotransmitter serotonin. And
you don't need to set aside hours
of your time, just 10 minutes a day
will see you feeling calmer, fitter and
more focused.

Choose your style

Hatha yoga – the physical form of yoga – comes in many different forms, and while these forms share much common ground, they each have a slightly different focus, some leaning towards physical benefits, others more spiritual ones. In this book, we've brought together five of the popular yoga styles so you can tailor your daily sessions to meet your needs.

● **Iyengar yoga** (p32) pays close attention to correct alignment, builds strength and creates a solid foundation for all other yoga styles.

● **Vinyasa yoga** (p50) has flowing sequences that are ideal for bringing more mindfulness into your life – you can move slowly to create a calming effect or up the tempo for more of a cardio workout.

● **Sivananda yoga** (p68) focuses on 12 poses and aims to help you achieve a state of optimal health and spiritual wellbeing through postures, relaxation, pranayama (breathing exercises) and meditation.

● **Yin yoga** (p86) works directly on your joints, tendons and ligaments, rather than your muscles so it's a great option to choose when you want to increase your flexibility.

● **Restorative yoga** (p106) is the one to turn to when you need to switch off completely from your busy life and rest and replenish your system.

What you need

Fitting yoga into your life every day takes a little planning to stop other commitments encroaching on your sessions.

■ **Time and place** Decide where and when you'll practise. It doesn't need to be the same time and place every day, although that will build an energy in the space you're using, helping you focus and making it easier for you to sink into a deeper place in meditation. Think about your regular commitments as well as when the other people in your house are around and possibly using your practice space. Then make a schedule, put it in your diary/phone calendar and treat it as a fixed date to help reinforce your commitment to stick to your goals.

■ **Clothing and kit** You don't need a lot of kit to practise yoga on a regular basis but a sticky mat is an essential to stop your feet slipping in poses such as Downward dog (p110). Comfortable clothing is a must – you need to be able to move freely – T-shirts and leggings are fine, but wear layers on top so you can remove them as your body heats up and replace them again for Savasana (relaxation). Avoid anything so loose that it rides up when you're in inverted poses, or so tight it feels restrictive. Specially bought props are tailor made for yoga, but you can easily substitute them with things around your home.

■ **Food and drink** It's best not to practise on a full stomach or you'll feel sluggish and uncomfortable, especially in poses that compress the abdomen, such as twists and forward bends, so plan your sessions at times when you won't have eaten a main meal in the previous two hours. You'll still need fuel, though, so have a banana, a handful of nuts or a yoghurt and some dates 30 minutes before you practise. Some people like to have a bottle of water to make sure they stay hydrated, especially for a demanding session such as a fast Vinyasa class; just make sure you take sips and not large gulps, as that can also feel uncomfortable on your stomach

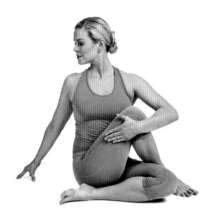

Tailor your sessions

● One of the beauties of a home practice is that you can tailor it to match your exact needs. As well as fitting it into your busy schedule, you can adapt the sessions to work with what else is going on in your life, rather than simply follow a teacher-led class. Want to go over the basics? Spend a few sessions working in depth with the Iyengar moves and sequence (p32). Need to increase your flexibility for another sport? Schedule in a couple of Yin sequences (p102) every week. Feeling burnt out from a heavy workload? Unwind after work with an evening Restorative session (p108) to soothe your nervous system and feel gently refreshed.

● You can tailor your warm-up to target whichever area of your body most needs freeing up – just ensure your spine is mobilised in a forwards and backwards plan (as in Cat/Cow, p20) as well as a sideways one (eg Shoulder stretch I, p23). You can also adapt the length of your session according to your available time.

● The Iyengar, Sivananda and Vinyasa asana sequences in this book can be done in just 10 minutes (you can practise the pranayama and meditations separately on busy days). But when you have more time to spend on your mat, you can make Iyengar and Sivananda more substantial sessions by spending longer in the poses.

How to breathe

In general, your breath instigates movement in yoga – you inhale as you unfold your body, lengthen your spine, open your chest or raise your arms. You exhale when you root into the ground, deepen into a forward fold or release into a twist. Most people breathe in quite a shallow way, but in yoga deep abdominal breathing will help you be more present in your practice.

Either sitting or lying, spend a few moments letting your breath settle, then take your hands and place them on your lower belly with your fingertips touching, heels of your hands out to the sides. Allow your breath to sink down and fill your belly as you inhale. Notice if you can feel your hands gently separating as your abdomen expands, and drawing together again as you exhale. After a few moments, slide your hands up to your side ribs. As you breathe in, notice if you can sense any movement beneath your hands. The gentle expansion of your ribs comes from the movement of your diaphragm as you inhale. Become aware of your ribs gently sinking back inwards as you exhale. Continue on your own for a few breaths, then slide your hands up to rest over your breastbone. Notice how your hands move as you take a few slow, deep breaths. In full abdominal breathing, aim to fill your belly, side ribs and upper chest in sequence as you inhale, emptying them in the reverse order as you exhale. This will help to bring a slow mindful quality to your yoga practice.

● You could also choose to repeat each pose in a sequence a second time; that way you can work on any areas you found a challenge on the first attempt or simply use it as an opportunity to sink more deeply into the asana, experiencing its qualities more deeply. Repeat the Vinyasa sequence twice through on less busy days, perhaps trying some of the moves with your eyes closed for a more meditative experience. Save the Yin and Restorative for those times when you won't feel rushed. It will be impossible to relax into the stretches and nourishing postures if you're constantly watching the clock.

QUICK TIPS

1 *Never push through pain*

It can worsen an inherent weakness or even be the catalyst for an injury. Forcing yourself to hold postures that your musculature isn't yet strong enough for can result in strains from which it can take weeks or months to recover. A dull ache is often a joint opening or muscle softening and is fine to work with – breathe into the tight area to help release it. But any hot, sharp or sudden pain should be avoided. Come out of the pose and try again another day, not moving so deeply into the pose. Trust your body, if something feels wrong to you, it probably is.

2 *Don't skip Savasana*

Many people think Savasana is the easy bit, where you just lie down and have a doze. In fact, BKS Iyengar once said Savasana is the most difficult pose of all. So few of us know how to relax deeply, but in Savasana we learn what complete relaxation means. It calms the nervous system, allows our body to come back to a state of equilibrium after our practice and, importantly, is the place where we absorb the benefits of the postures.

3 *Be kind to yourself*

It's not unusual to experience strong emotions during yoga, especially as you develop a regular practice. It may be a feeling of strength, empowerment or joy, but equally you may feel vulnerable, sad or fearful. Your body stores emotional memories and, as you begin to open and release your muscles, emotions are sometimes released. If this happens to you, trust your instincts and follow what you need. You may wish to stop and rest in Savasana, and simply allow the emotion to run its natural course, or you may want to carry on with your sequence, simply being a witness to the emotion but not identifying with it. You can also reflect on your experience during your meditation sessions. The important thing is to not judge your experience – just let it be part of the journey you are on – because, in time, you'll come to understand it more.

> *You can adapt the sessions to work with what is going on in your life, rather than simply follow a teacher-led class*

21 WAYS TO DO

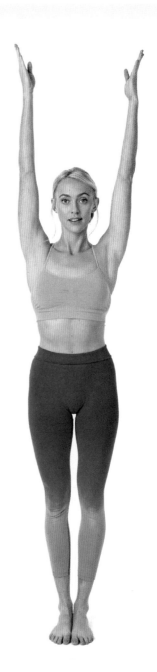

You already know how good yoga can make you feel – calmer, more energised, focused, strong and flexible – so imagine the difference a daily session could make to your life. We know that finding the time to get on your mat every day can be a challenge, so we've put together these simple tips to help make your yoga dreams a reality.

1 Make a commitment
It's easier to stick to a goal if you make it a conscious decision. Set aside time to understand why you want to practise yoga more regularly. Reflect on some of the things that might sabotage your attempts, what you can put in place to meet those challenges and any other ways you can support yourself in your new direction. It's helpful to get into a meditative space before you begin, so close your eyes and spend five minutes calming your mind with some deep abdominal breathing. When you've finished your reflections, writing them down will help you connect back to them when needed.

2 Indulge for a moment
Remind yourself why you love yoga. Remember the person you are when you practise yoga, and get on your mat and do your favourite pose. Play music, light a candle, open the windows and let the fresh air in - enjoy the moment, luxuriate in it, be totally absorbed by it, and the next time you're tempted to drop a session tune into these feelings, and let yourself experience them again.

3 Be realistic
If you know that even a short daily asana session isn't possible at the moment, plan a schedule that is doable. Maybe try two asana sessions a week and a five-minute meditation or pranayama practice on the remaining days.

4 Make it physical
One way to help reinforce a decision is to have a physical representation of the commitment. Buy yourself that yoga mat you've always fancied, invest in some new yoga clothes, get yourself a couple of yoga props. Creating something physical out of what was once just a thought will remind you of the promise you've made to yourself and will ground your decision in reality.

5 Prioritise
Sometimes we have to let something go if we want to incorporate a new activity or commitment into our lives. Do you really need to watch that box set? Could you spend less time on social media? Be clear on what matters more to you, then act accordingly.

6 Take five
When you're thinking of skipping a session, changing your surroundings can help you make the best choice. Go into another room, close your eyes, take a few deep breaths then ask yourself what you most need now – to get on your mat or to do something else – then follow what your intuition says.

yoga every day

7 Reignite your passion
Do a workshop with a visiting teacher, go on a yoga holiday, set yourself a new goal or a seven-day challenge or sign up for a free session on one of the streaming sites such as ekhartyoga.com or doyouyoga.com.

8 Move up the list
Are your needs at the bottom of your to-do list? Do you fall in with your partner's timetable? Does your flatmate decide what happens in your shared space? Is your boss's agenda obscuring your own? Making space for yoga will help you skilfully negotiate all of these situations so that you have more of a voice in your own life.

9 Mix it up Doing the same routine, in the same place, every day can leave you stuck and uninspired. Varying how, when and where you practise will help you stay committed. Schedule in morning, after work and bedtime sessions; if you have space in your home, follow the sun – practising in one room for the morning light, another to catch the sunset; if you have a garden (or a nearby park), practise outside in warmer weather, buddy up and have a yoga date with a friend - one time at her place, the next at yours.

10 Check in Ask yourself why you're missing your sessions. Be honest, don't accept the first thing that comes into your head, it's likely to be a quick excuse. Close your eyes, tune into your intuition and understand the deeper reason you've gone back on your commitment. Then, ask that place of wisdom for one thing you could do to help you make space for yourself again.

11 Slow down One of the reasons we do yoga is to calm a busy mind and have space to breathe. Try typing slowly, washing the dishes slowly or preparing the evening meal slowly. The minute you stop rushing your shoulders will drop and you'll sink into a more yogic frame of mind.

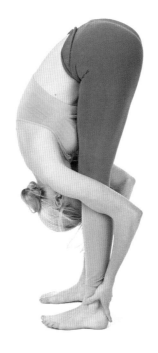

Go bite size

If you're still struggling to fit in a yoga session, try some of these simple check-ins, so you still connect with your yoga journey every day.

12 Do a few rounds of Sun or Moon salutes.

13 Practise one pose a day.

14 Play yoga games with your children.

15 Practise deep abdominal breathing at your computer.

16 Do a five-minute meditation or breathing practice before you get up in the morning, during your commute or in the supermarket queue.

17 Stand in Tree pose while the kettle boils.

18 Do a simple twist or shoulder stretch in your office chair every couple of hours.

19 Take three deep breaths before every decision, each time you walk through a doorway or see a traffic light.

20 Do some hip openers while you're watching the news on TV.

21 Stream an inspiring yoga class, dharma talk or chant during your commute.

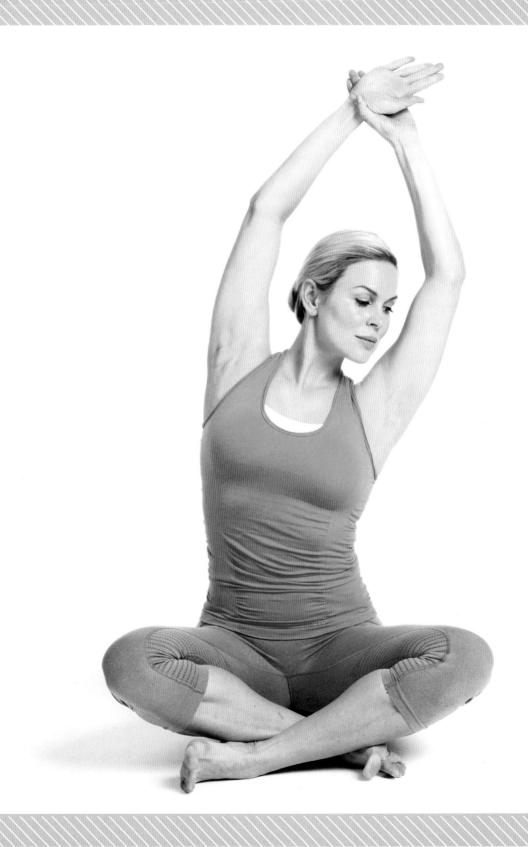

Get moving

Now that you have **the basics** in place it's time to start moving. In this section, we show you how to prepare your body for your practice with a series of **warm-ups** to mobilise your spine, open your hips and release your shoulders so that you stay safe in your sessions. Don't be tempted to skip this section as warm **muscles** will prevent injury and help you get into the poses more easily. You'll also find a selection of four Sun and Moon salutes you can use to tailor your **daily practice** to suit your energy level and goals. Sun salute I is a gentle introduction to the form, while Sun salute II is a more challenging version where you jump into poses to **build upper body** and **core strength**. Try the Moon salutes when you want a more inward practice and to soothe your body at the end of the day.

WARM-up

Warming your muscles and gently releasing your joints in preparation for your yoga session is crucial for preventing injury. It boosts your circulation so muscles receive more oxygen and energy for the demands of your session, and stimulates the production of synovial fluid, the protective liquid inside the joint capsule that cushions and lubricates your joints. But a yoga warm-up does more than that: it helps you transition from your busy day to a more reflective space where you can tune into your needs and the deeper aspects of yourself. As you concentrate on your breath, body and mind, the outside world grows quiet, your worries subside and you can focus on nourishing yourself for the next hour or so. Let's begin.

Awaken your spine

If you do no other warm-up, always loosen your vertebral column before your yoga practice. Moving your spine in all its planes of movement — forwards and backwards, sideways and rotational (with twists) — will help keep it healthy, flexible and strong.

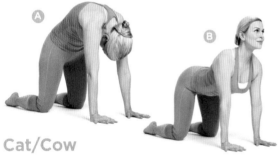

Cat/Cow

Cat/Cow mobilises your spine forwards and backwards. From all-fours, inhale, then, as you exhale, root through the base of your index fingers and thumbs and the tops of your toes as you release your head and tailbone to the floor and lift your spine towards the ceiling into Cat. On your next inhale, tilt your tailbone up and release your spine down into a backbend. Draw your shoulders down your back, take your chest forwards and up and raise your head into Cow. Alternate between Cat and Cow, instigating the movement from your pelvis and following your breath. Move vertebra by vertebra in a fluid way. You can explore free-form Cat/Cow and move spontaneously; push your hips back to elongate your spine, move your right then left buttock to the side to stretch your oblique muscles, roll your shoulders and circle your neck.

Child's pose

Kneel on your mat and take your knees wide, big toes together, heels falling out to the sides. Lower your buttocks onto the soles of your feet and rest your palms on your thighs. Inhale as you root into your sitting bones to lengthen your spine. On an exhale, walk your hands forwards, as you lower your torso between your thighs, lowering your head to rest your forehead on the floor, a block or bolster. Or, rest on one cheek, drawing your shoulders away from your ears. Close your eyes, then take your hands beside your hips, palms facing upwards. Slide your shoulder blades down your back and your tailbone towards your heels. Breathe deeply and evenly into your back body for up to five minutes, turning your head halfway through if you're resting on your cheek. You can use Child's pose whenever you need to rest.

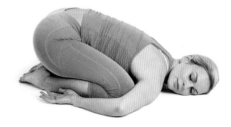

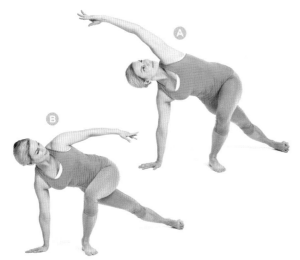

Tiger stretch

From Cat, inhale and stretch your right leg back and up, bending your knee and pointing your toes towards your head into Tiger (A). Pause, then, as you exhale, bring your right knee towards your chest as you arc your spine upwards (B). Moving in time with your breath, repeat a few times, then lower and repeat on the other side.

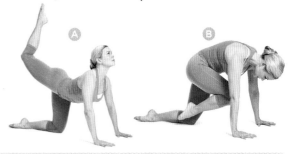

Nectar of the flowing moon

Step into a lunge, with your left foot forwards, hands either side of your foot. Take your weight onto your right hand, pivot clockwise on your front heel, turning your toes out 90 degrees. At the same time, pivot on your back toes, taking your heel to the right, so you rest on the outer edge of your back foot. Ground through your right hand, inhale and bring your left arm forwards and alongside your ear and look towards your left hand (A). Keep your legs active, and root through your feet to lift your chest and lengthen the left side of your body, from your foot to your fingertips. Exhale, sweep your left arm alongside your top hip and gaze at your fingertips (B). Continue moving between these poses for a few rounds, arcing a little deeper into a backbend on each inhale, softening as your exhale. Exhale to lower then repeat on the other side.

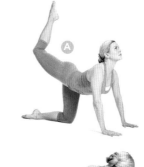

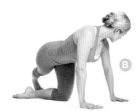

Side stretch

From Tiger (A), inhale and extend your right leg and rest your toes outside your left foot to lengthen and open your right body into Side stretch. Gaze over your left shoulder to look at your right foot (B). Take a few breaths into your right ribs, then raise your right foot, place it out to the side and point your toes. Raise your right arm alongside your ear and lift into Side gate (C). Feel the stretch from your right toes to your right fingertips. Take five deep breaths into your right ribs, exhale to lower and repeat on the other side.

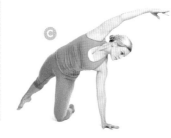

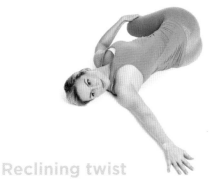

Reclining twist

Lying on your back, hug both knees to your chest, using your forearms to bring your knees in close and draw your shoulder blades down your back. Take a few breaths here, then exhale as you release both knees over to the left, resting your left hand on your right knee to gently deepen the stretch. Extend your right arm to the side and, if comfortable, gently turn your head to look to the right. Breathe deeply into your right side, enjoying the stretch for 10 deep breaths, then slowly inhale back to centre and repeat on the other side. To facilitate this twist and maintain good alignment of your spine, before you begin, lift your buttocks and shift them slightly to the left before twisting to the right, and vice versa.

Loosen your hips

Freedom in your pelvis influences freedom of movement in your spine, and increasing flexibility in your hips will support many yoga poses, including Warrior II, Triangle, Wide-legged standing or seated forward fold and Butterfly. If your hips are tight, try to do Butterfly each day, supporting your knees with bolsters if needed.

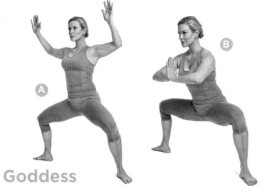

Goddess

Step your feet wide, toes turned out 45 degrees and ground through your big toes and outer edges of your feet. Inhale, then exhale to bend your knees over your middle toes, keeping your spine vertical. If your knees fall inwards, bring your toes in slightly or step your feet closer together. Lengthen your tailbone towards the floor and draw your belly button towards your spine. Inhale as you circle your arms to the sides to shoulder height, then bend your elbows 90 degrees to take your forearms to vertical. Face your palms forwards (A). Exhale as you sink deeper into the pose. Breathe deeply for five to 10 breaths, feeling the grounded strength of your legs, the gentle opening of your hips and heart. When your hips feel more open, lower into High garland (B).

Half squat

From Crescent (p56), place both hands on the mat inside your right foot. Walk your hands to your right as you pivot on the ball of your left foot and heel of your right foot to face the long side of the mat. Sit back on your left heel and take your left knee out to the side, pointing your right toes up. Root through your left toes as you inhale to lift your torso, shoulder blades sliding down your spine. Bring your hands into prayer position, focusing on a fixed point to aid your balance, or put your hands on the floor. Breathe deeply for three to five breaths. Lower your hands to the floor, walk them to your right, transfer your weight to your right foot, and repeat on the other side.

Eye of the needle

Lie on your back and rest your left ankle on your right thigh. Thread your left hand between your thighs and interlace your fingers behind your right knee (A). If your hands don't reach, wrap a strap around your right thigh (B). Use your arms to draw your right knee towards your chest as you press your left forearm into your left thigh to open your left hip. Take five deep breaths here, then repeat on the other side.

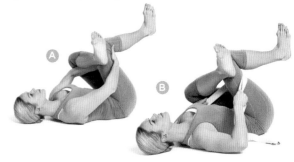

Reclining hand-to-toe pose

Lie on your back and hug your right knee into your chest. Wrap a strap around the ball of your right foot and, on an inhale, straighten your leg. Exhale as you rotate your hip outwards and lower your leg to the side. If necessary, use your left hand to push your left hip onto the floor; otherwise, extend your left arm out to the side. Beginners: if your lower back comes off the floor, bend your left knee and place your foot flat on the floor. Take five deep breaths, inhale to bring your leg back to centre and exhale to gently lower it. Repeat on the other side.

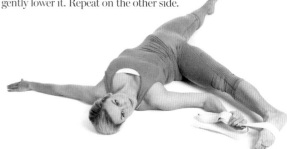

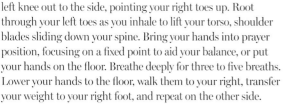

Stretch your shoulders

Loosening tight shoulders will help you in any pose where your arms reach overhead, such as High lunge, Downward dog and Wheel. And because muscles in your arms link to your lower back, increasing shoulder mobility will help with backbends, too.

Flowing half squat

From Half squat (p22), with a flowing breath, let your upper body cascade forwards as you transfer your weight from one foot (A) to the other (B), bending one knee deeply and straightening the other. Keep your spine long, release your neck and let your upper body and arms move in a flowing motion. Alternate between your right and left sides, breathing freely and trailing your arms and hands on the floor in a large figure of eight.

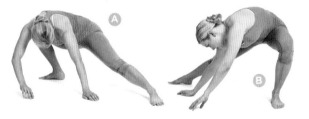

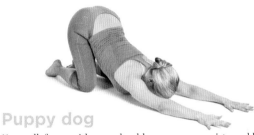

Puppy dog

From all-fours, with your shoulders over your wrists and hips over your knees, lie your toes flat on the floor and walk your hands forwards a hand's-length or two. Inhale, then exhale and root through your hands as you take your hips back to lengthen your spine. Walk your hands forwards a bit more to keep your thighs vertical, then, with your fingers spread, lower your head to the floor or a folded blanket. Relax your neck, take five deep breaths into your back body, then walk your hands in and come back to kneeling.

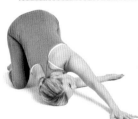

Thread the needle

As well as increasing mobility in your shoulders, this warm-up is also a gentle twist, so you can use it to awaken your spine as well. From all-fours, with your shoulders over your wrists and hips over your knees, inhale and raise your right arm out to the side. On an exhale, slide your arm beneath your torso, palm facing up, extending your hand under your left arm and out to the side. Take your left hand forwards a few inches, then press into the floor to lift your left shoulder , lower your head to the floor and deepen the twist. Exhale to release, then repeat on the other side.

Shoulder stretch I

From a sitting position, inhale and take your arms overhead, fingers interlaced, palms facing the ceiling. Take hold of your right wrist with your left hand, inhale and root through your sitting bones, using your left hand to lift your right arm higher. Feel your spine elongate. As you exhale, draw your right hand over to the left, taking care not to let your body lean forwards or backwards. Inhale, root down and lengthen a little more, then fold further to the left on an exhale. Take one more deep breath, then inhale back to centre and repeat on the other side. Lower both arms on an exhale.

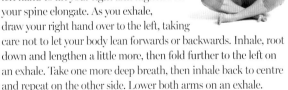

Shoulder stretch II

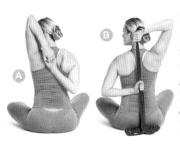

In a sitting position, inhale and raise your left arm to the side, shoulder height. Rotate your palm to face the ceiling, then keep raising your arm until your upper arm is close to your ear. As you exhale, fold your forearm to rest your palm on the centre of your upper back, elbow pointing up. Inhale and raise your right arm to the side, about 45 degrees. Turn your palm to face the back of the room, bend your elbow, place the back of your hand between your shoulder blades, and hold the fingertips of your left hand (A). If your hands don't connect, use a strap (B). Take three to five deep breaths into your belly, rooting through your sitting bones. Release on an exhale and repeat on the other side.

Surya namaskar I

● Sun salutes awaken your spine in a forwards and backwards plane, creating heat in your body to support the poses you will be doing in your main practice. They're also a great mini sequence to use on a daily basis when you don't have time for a longer session.
● Move slowly initially to gently warm your muscles, then work at the pace that's right for your body today. Moving faster will awaken and energise you, moving slower will heighten your sensitivity and leave you feeling calmer and more grounded
● On your first circuit, lead with your right foot, taking five deep breaths into your belly for each pose. This will help to bring you into a mindful connection with your body and give you time to refine your alignment. Once you come back to Mountain pose (p36), repeat the sequence again, this time leading with your left leg. This forms one round of the Sun salutation. On the following rounds, using the breathing pattern suggested below will enable you to make the sequence one continuous flow.

The sequence

1 Mountain pose (p36)
Inhale, root through your feet and take your arms out to the sides and overhead to...

2 Extended mountain pose (p36)
Arch your back slightly, then exhale and take your arms to the sides and down into...

3 Standing forward fold (p82)
Inhale as you step your right leg back to...

4 Crescent (p56)
Exhale and step your left foot back to...

5 Plank (p58)
Pause the breath as you lower your knees and chest to the floor, and then your abdomen into...

6 Caterpillar
Inhale into...

7 Cobra (p77)
Exhale and root through your hands to lift back into...

8 Downward dog (p110)
Take five deep breaths here 'walking the dog' by bending one knee then the other, and focus on lifting your tailbone up and back to lengthen your spine. Inhale as you step your right foot forwards into...

9 Crescent (p56)
Exhale and step your right foot back into...

10 Standing forward fold (p82)
Inhale, taking your arms out to the side and overhead to...

11 Extended mountain pose (p36)
Exhale your arms out to the side and to prayer, then back into...

12 Mountain pose (p36)
Repeat, leading with your left leg. This is one round.

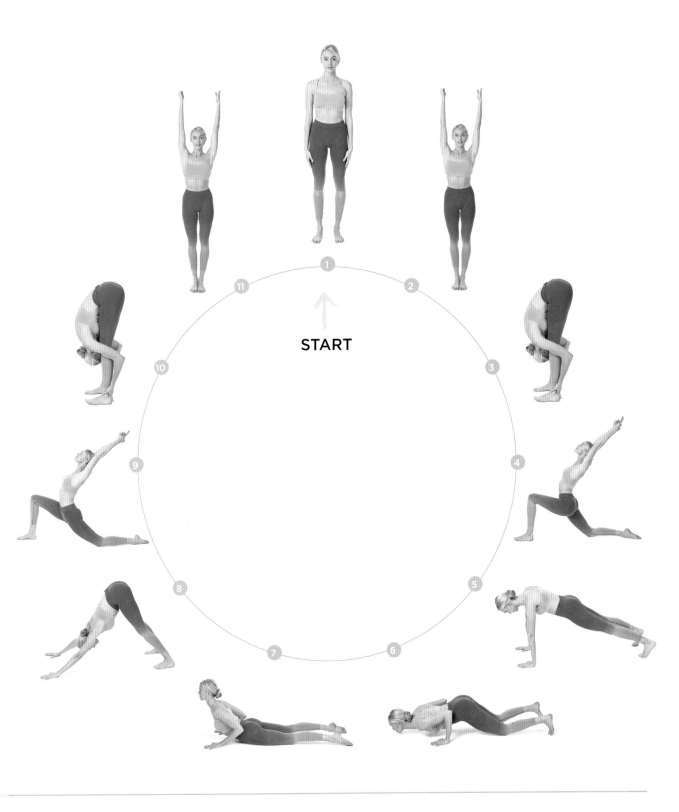

START

Surya namaskar II

● Once you're comfortable with Sun salute I you can begin to incorporate other moves into the sequence. There are several variations to Sun salutes, and this challenging one is comes from the Iyengar school of yoga. It strengthens your arms, legs, core and back. If you're new to Four-limbed staff pose, you may prefer to replace it with High plank while you build up your strength.

● This Sun salute is generally practised relatively fast, following the breathing pattern below, but always listen to your body and follow what it needs on the day. For example, if you're low in energy you may prefer to step between postures instead of jumping, but when you do jump, aim to land as lightly as possible on your feet. Over time and with regular practice you'll build sufficient strength to slowly 'float' instead of jump between the postures. This is a beautiful expression of poise and control in your practice. Using Ujjayi breathing (p35) will help to give you the power and energy you need.

The sequence

1 Mountain pose
(p36)
Root through your feet, inhale and take your arms overhead into...

2 Extended mountain pose
(p36)
Exhale as you hinge from your hips and fold into...

3 Standing forward fold (p82)
Bend your knees deeply, inhale, exhale and jump back into...

4 Four-limbed staff pose
Inhale into...

5 Downward dog
(p110)
Exhale into...

6 Four-limbed staff pose
Inhale into...

7 Cobra (or Upward facing dog) (p77)
Exhale into...

8 Four-limbed staff pose
Inhale to...

9 Downward dog
(p110)
Bend your knees deeply, inhale and float or jump forwards into ...

10 Standing forward fold (p82)
Inhale and come back up to...

11 Extended mountain pose
(p36)
Exhale and lower your arms into...

12 Mountain pose
(p36)

Tip

When transitioning between Four-limbed staff pose (Chaturanga) and Cobra (poses 6 and 7) give your toes a thorough workout by rolling over your toes from curled under in Chaturanga to resting on the tops of your toes in Cobra.

EXPERIENCED YOGIS
If you're familiar with this sequence, you may like to use Upward Dog pose instead of Cobra, resting on your hands and tops of your feet only.

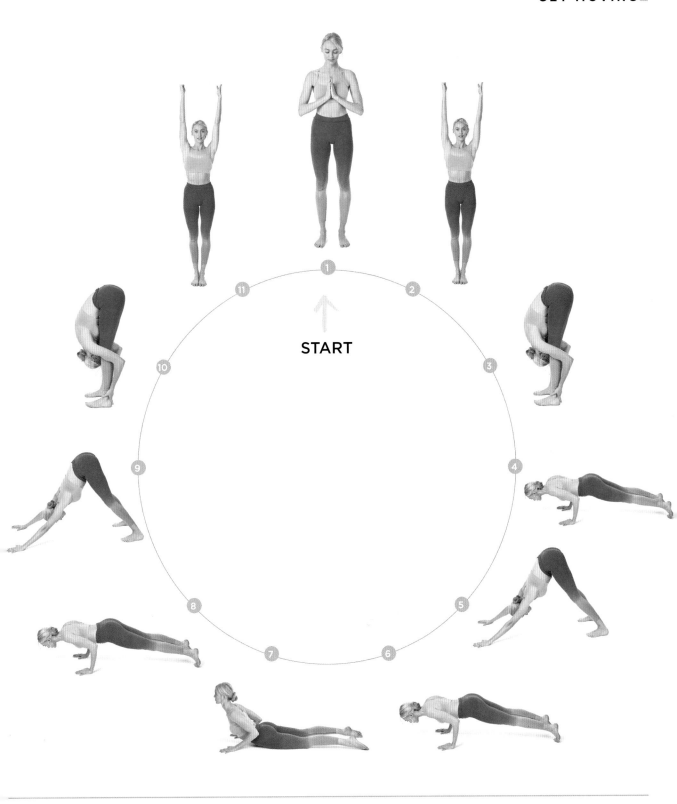

START

Chandra namaskar I

Moon salutes are the ideal practice for those times when you're low in energy, menstruating or looking for a soft slow sequence to get your body moving. Allow each pose to flow into the next using your breath to support you, following the breathing pattern below for two or three rounds.

The sequence

1 Mountain pose (p36)
Inhale, and take your arms out to the side and overhead, then exhale into...

2 Extended mountain pose with side bend (p36)
Extend to the left, then inhale to centre and exhale to the right. Inhale back up and step sideways with your left foot. Exhale into...

3 Goddess (p22)
Inhale. Turn your left foot out 90 degrees, and your right foot in slightly, and exhale into...

4 Triangle (p83)
Inhale, then exhale as you lower your right hand and turn both hips to the left, pivoting on your back foot, to come into...

5 Pyramid (p41)
Inhale, then exhale as you lower your right knee to the floor. Inhale into...

6 Crescent (p56)
Exhale and lower your hands to the floor and turn to your right into...

7 Half squat (p22)
Inhale into prayer, then lower your hands and exhale into...

8 Garland (p81)
Inhale into prayer, then lower your hands and exhale into...

9 Half squat (p22)
Inhale into prayer, then exhale as you lower your hands and turn to your right, lower your left knee and inhale into...

10 Crescent (p56)
Exhale, lower your hands, then inhale and rise into...

11 Pyramid (p41)
Exhale, then inhale, taking your left arm in a large arc into...

12 Triangle (p83)
Exhale, then inhale to come up and exhale into...

13 Goddess (p22)
Inhale as you step your feet together, exhale as you bring your hands to prayer. Inhale into...

14 Extended mountain pose with side bend (p36)
Exhale to the left, inhale to centre, exhale to the right, inhale back to centre, and exhale into...

15 Mountain pose (p36)
Pause, then repeat, leading with the opposite leg.

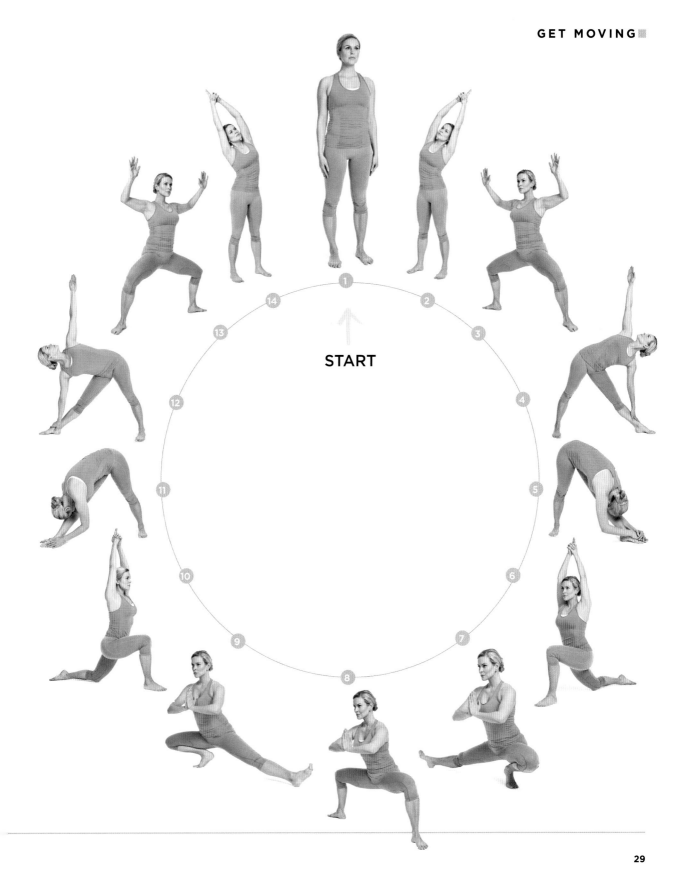

START

MOON SALUTE II
Chandra namaskar II

Once you're familiar with Moon salute I (p28), try this freer form, which lets you express more how your body feels in the moment. Tune inwards and sense what the pose feels like. Do you need to extend more to feel you're fully stretching your spine? Would moving slowly deepen your experience? Do you need the energising boost of a faster flow? Try closing your eyes: what difference does it make? As you learn to be guided by your experience, you can tailor your practice so it becomes like medicine for your mind and body.

The sequence

1 Mountain pose
Stand with your hands softly at your heart, palms facing up and little fingers touching.

2 Heart-opening pose
Inhale, circle your hands out to the side and, on an exhale, rest them on your sacrum. Inhale, root through your feet and lift through your chest into a backbend.

3 Lunar standing forward fold
Exhale as you fold from your hips. Keep your knees soft and let your chest drape over your thighs. Rest your hands on your mat, palms up. Inhale, step your left foot straight back then turn your front foot out 90 degrees and swivel onto the outside edge of your back foot.

4 Nectar of the moon I
Inhale to bring your right arm alongside your ear. Ground through your left hand to lift and open your chest.

5 Nectar of the moon II
Exhale as you arc your right arm around towards your back foot. Move between your left and right feet a few times then, finishing by your left foot. Place your hands either side of your foot and pivot to your left.

6-7 Spontaneous flowing half squat
Move between 6 and 7 three times, then, from 7, pivot on your feet and walk your hands round to your left so you face the short side of the mat.

8 Downward dog
Bring your feet hip-distance apart, lift your hips to the ceiling, ground your hands, Exhale into...

9 Puppy dog
Rest for a few breaths, then inhale as you come forwards to lower onto your stomach. Exhale. Inhale into...

10-12 Spontaneous flowing cobra
Rise up and down a couple of times, allowing your upper spine and shoulders to move in a fluid spontaneous way. Come up into full Cobra. Lower to the floor on an exhale, rest for a couple of breaths, then inhale and into...

13 Bliss-filled downward dog
Move as freely as your body needs to for a few breaths, maybe slowly 'walking the dog' or circling your hips. Pause, then inhale and raise your left leg into...

14 Downward dog splits
Exhale to lower your left leg. Inhale and raise your right leg, then exhale as you bring it forwards into...

15 Lunar standing forward fold
Inhale and uncurl into...

16 Heart-opening pose
Root through your feet as you lift into your heart and crown. Pause, imagining you're being bathed in moonlight, then exhale into...

17 Mountain pose
Pause, tune into how you feel. When you're ready, repeat the sequence on the other side, stepping back with your right leg.

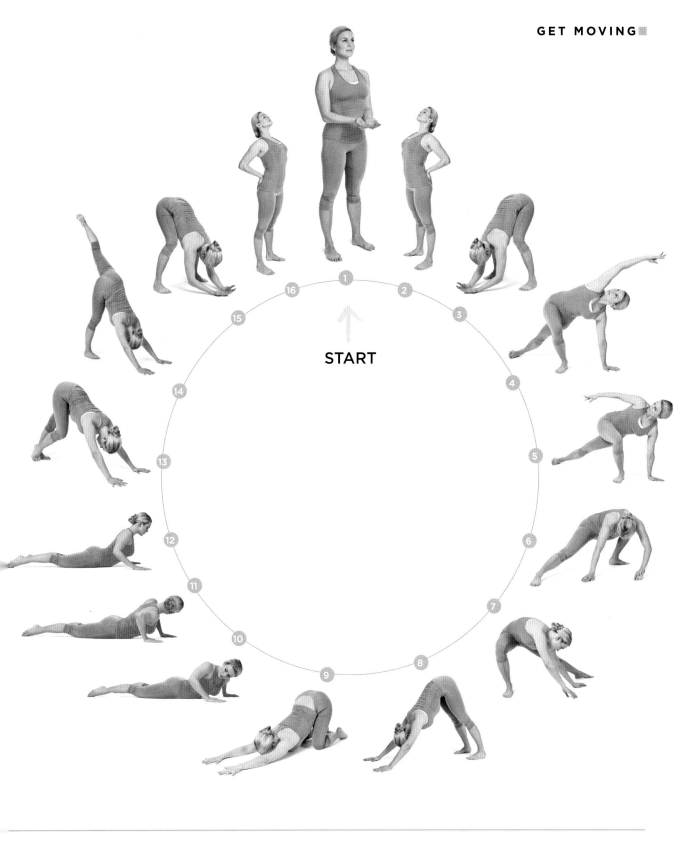

START

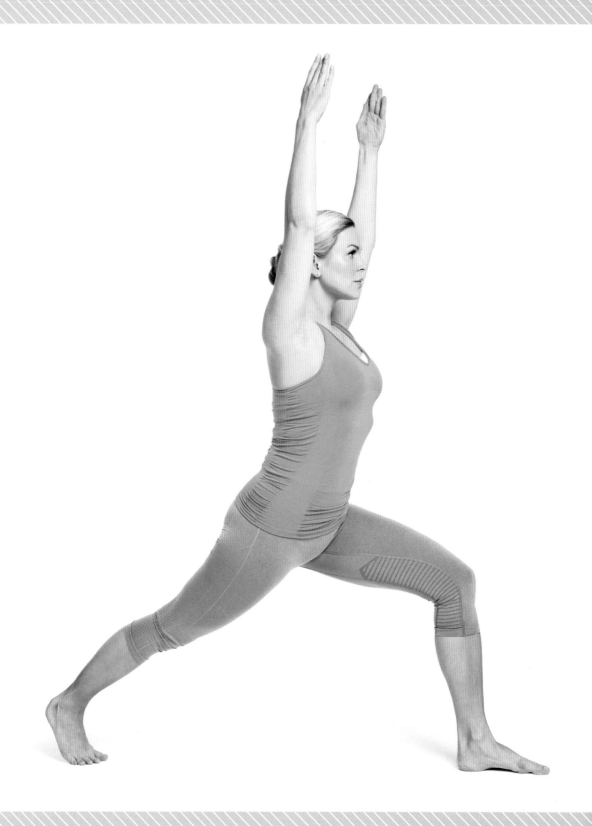

Iyengar

Welcome to the main aspect of your yoga practice: the *postures*. We begin our journey with the Iyengar style of yoga, as it has a strong focus on accurate alignment and will teach you valuable *skills and principles* that will help you maximise the benefits you gain from your sessions. What's more, these alignment guides apply to most yoga styles, perhaps with the exception of Yin and Restorative, so they will stand you in good stead no matter what style you decide to focus on. When you're *learning* allow plenty of time for the standing postures, as they will help you build strength and stamina. Mountain pose (p36), in particular, will teach you key *alignment* points that are repeated in all standing poses. Staff pose (p43), meanwhile, forms the basis of the seated postures, so spend time absorbing the *guidelines* here too.

INTRODUCTION TO
Iyengar

Founder of Iyengar yoga, BSK Iyengar, made an enormous contribution to the world of yoga, systemising more than 200 asanas and pranayama (breathing) techniques, and bringing them to the West from India. Although correct form was vital to Iyengar, he's perhaps best known for introducing props – such as chairs, cushions, blocks, bolsters and straps – into his classes, so that everyone could experience the benefits of yoga, regardless of their ability. It was through these modifications that Iyengar developed a system of therapeutic applications for yoga, seen most clearly in his book *Yoga: the Path to Holistic Health* (Dorling Kindersley, £25). Whether you're suffering from migraine, acne, asthma, sciatica, depression or menstrual irregularities, Iyengar has a sequence of poses that can bring relief.

But his form of yoga went far deeper than just the physical postures; pranayama and meditation are combined to unite 'the individual self with the universal self', he said. And the result? 'The primary aim of yoga is to restore the mind to simplicity and peace, and to free it from confusion and distress,' he said. 'The practice of yoga fills up the reservoirs of hope and optimism within you.'

> *The primary aim of yoga is to restore the mind to simplicity and peace, and to free it from confusion and distress*

BEFORE YOU BEGIN

● Feel free to use any props you need to help you find the correct alignment in the pose. Rather than think of yourself as being a beginner for using a prop, know that you are intelligently supporting your body to maximise your experience of the posture. It could be the configuration of your anatomy, rather than a lack of flexibility, that makes a posture a challenge for you. Sit on a block or bolster if your back rounds in seated postures; use a block as an extension of your arms in poses such as Pyramid (p41), Camel (p60) or Half moon (p59), and a strap around your legs in Seated forward fold (p76).

● Aim to breathe evenly in each of the postures, taking your breath down into your abdomen.

● If you want to support yourself even more, try Ujayi breathing. Also known as Victorious breath, Ujjayi works on every cell in your body, boosts your energy and helps to focus your mind.

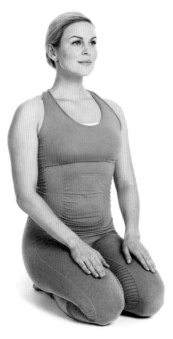

Pranayama

UJJAYI BREATHING

■ Lying in Relaxation pose (p47), close your eyes and spend a moment or two allowing your mind and breath to settle. Then, on your next inhalation, imagine a fine golden thread of light filtering down from the sky and entering the front of your throat. Sense it travel to the back of your throat and, as you exhale, feel the light float up from the back of your throat to the front and to the sky again. Continue breathing in this way for a few minutes, allowing a softness and stillness to settle around you.

■ Next, come to a comfortable seated position, become still once more, then continue drawing the thread of light towards your throat, this time from the horizon rather than the sky. Let a sense of quietness envelop you for a few more moments, then gently let your breath return to normal.

■ Finally, gently open your lips and breathe in and out through your mouth, this time making a soft 'haaa' sound as you do so, which will slightly close your throat, the key action of Ujjayi. Continue for a few more moments, breathing gently, so that only someone sitting close to you would hear the 'haaa' sound. Then gently let it go and softly open your eyes.

Meditation

DHYANA

■ This practice is all about withdrawal: quietening your senses and going deeply inwards. At first, some of the guidelines may seem difficult or even impossible to achieve, but if you remain open, have the intention of fulfilling them – or even imagine you're doing them – over time your sensitivity will grow and you'll begin to experience the subtleties they refer to.

■ Sit in a comfortable position, gently close your eyes and bring your hands into prayer position at the centre of your chest, thumbs pointing to the base of your sternum, fingers pointing away from your chest. Relax your arms so that your elbows release down towards your waist.

■ Soften your eyeballs and withdraw your gaze inwards. Withdraw your hearing from the outer portion of your ear. Withdraw your breath from the inside surface of your nostrils, and withdraw sensation from the front of your tongue. Keep breathing softy and gently, allowing your breath to become subtler and subtler.

■ Withdraw your flesh away from your skin surface, your skull from your scalp and your brain from your skull. Rest your attention on your back brain at the base of your skull.

■ Reconnect to your sight and hearing and the sensation of your tongue. Gather them together and bring them to the back surface of your sternum at the base, which is said to be your heart centre. Let your thumbs merge with your heart centre and your fingertips reach out and merge with the universe.

■ When you feel ready, release your hands and lie in Relaxation pose (p47) for a few minutes to absorb your experience, then gently open your eyes and come up to sitting.

MOUNTAIN POSE
Tadasana

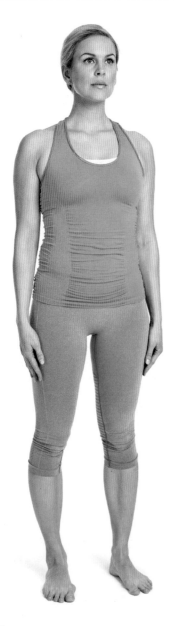

● Place your feet shoulder-width apart, inner edges parallel. Balance your weight evenly over each foot, spread your toes and root through the base of your big and little toes. Lift your inner arches by drawing your ankles away from each other.

● Align your knees over your ankles and your pelvis over your knees. Relax your buttocks and allow your tail and sitting bones to release to the floor. Breathe deeply and evenly.

● Draw your navel towards your spine and release your shoulders down your back. Let your arms hang loosely at your sides, then gently extend through to your fingertips. Release and lengthen the back of your neck.

● As you inhale, ground through your feet and feel the corresponding lift in your spine as you lengthen through to the crown of your head, maintaining the length in your torso when you exhale. Let your breath be gentle, feeling the length and lightness of each in-breath, and a sense of grounding and stability on the out-breath. Rest in the pose for up to 20 to 30 seconds.

VARIATION
Extended mountain pose
From Mountain pose (above) inhale and root though your feet as you lift your waist out of your hips to lengthen your spine. At the same time, turn your palms outwards and extend your arms in a large circle out to the sides of your body and overhead so they are pointing to the ceiling. Ground through your feet as you reach through to your fingertips, drawing your navel to your spine, and your shoulder blades down your back. Keep your gaze soft.

Good for:

- *Grounding and calming*
- *Improving your posture*
- *Improving alignment of your body*
- *Countering degenerative effects of ageing on your spine, legs and feet*

Iyengar says...

66 Practising this pose gives rise to a sense of firmness, strength, stillness and steadiness. 99

CHAIR POSE

Utkatasana

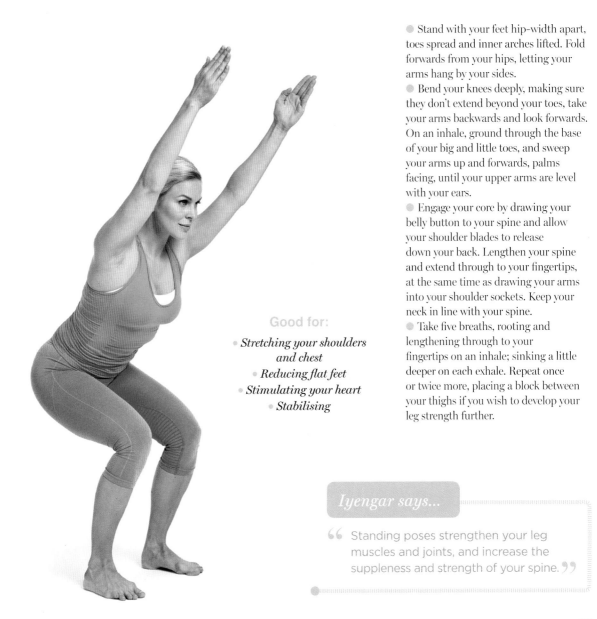

Good for:

- *Stretching your shoulders and chest*
- *Reducing flat feet*
- *Stimulating your heart*
- *Stabilising*

● Stand with your feet hip-width apart, toes spread and inner arches lifted. Fold forwards from your hips, letting your arms hang by your sides.

● Bend your knees deeply, making sure they don't extend beyond your toes, take your arms backwards and look forwards. On an inhale, ground through the base of your big and little toes, and sweep your arms up and forwards, palms facing, until your upper arms are level with your ears.

● Engage your core by drawing your belly button to your spine and allow your shoulder blades to release down your back. Lengthen your spine and extend through to your fingertips, at the same time as drawing your arms into your shoulder sockets. Keep your neck in line with your spine.

● Take five breaths, rooting and lengthening through to your fingertips on an inhale; sinking a little deeper on each exhale. Repeat once or twice more, placing a block between your thighs if you wish to develop your leg strength further.

Iyengar says...

" Standing poses strengthen your leg muscles and joints, and increase the suppleness and strength of your spine. "

WARRIOR II
Virabhadrasana II

From standing, step your feet wide, turning your left foot out 90 degrees and your right foot in 15 degrees. Align your left heel with your right heel or, for beginners, your right instep. Spread your toes and root through your big and little toes and the outside edge of your right foot.

With your weight balanced evenly between both feet, your pelvis in neutral and facing the long side of your mat, inhale to raise your arms to the sides, palms facing the floor. Lengthen from your centre to beyond your fingertips.

On an exhale, bend your left leg to take your knee directly over your ankle, keeping a micro-bend in your right leg. Keep your spine vertical. If you find yourself leaning forwards, extend your back hand towards the back of the mat.

Breathing evenly, draw your navel to your spine, open your chest and slide your shoulders down your spine. If comfortable, turn your head to gaze along your front arm, beyond your middle finger.

Rest in the pose for 30 seconds, drawing your inner thighs together and feeling how the strength of your lower body brings a freedom to your upper body. When you feel ready, exhale, gently lower your hands and step your feet together.

Pause for a moment before repeating on the other side.

Good for:

- *Increasing focus and determination*
- *Strengthening your legs*
- *Grounding*
- *Easing lower back pain*

VARIATIONS
Reverse warrior

From Warrior II, inhale as you slide your back arm down your back thigh, and raise your front arm overhead, gently arching your spine laterally. Root your feet down and lift your torso up on each inhale, feeling your side body open, and, as you exhale, arc a little further into the backbend. Take five breaths, then change sides.

Iyengar says...

"Warrior II exercises your limbs and torso vigorously, reducing stiffness in your neck and shoulders. It also makes your knee and hip joints more flexible."

EXTENDED SIDE ANGLE
Uttitha parsvakonasana

● Step your feet wide and turn your right foot out 90 degrees, your left foot in 15 degrees. Align your right heel to your left instep and root through your toes and outer edge of your left foot.

● Balance your weight evenly between both feet, inhale and raise your arms to the sides, shoulder height.

● Exhale, bend your right knee over your ankle, keeping a micro-bend in your left leg as you take your right forearm to your thigh and your left hand to your left hip.

● Tilt your tailbone towards your back heel and rotate your chest upwards and open. Then, on an inhale, sweep your left arm overhead and alongside your ear, palm facing down. (If you feel comfortable here, you can deepen the stretch by placing your right hand on the floor outside your front foot.)

● Ground through the outer edge of your back foot to lengthen your entire left side body, from your foot right through to your left fingertips. Gaze at the floor or, if comfortable for your neck, your upper hand.

● Breathe into your belly for 20 to 30 seconds, savouring the stretch, then when ready, exhale and return to standing. Pause, and repeat on the other side.

Good for:

● *Grounding*

● *Strengthening your legs*

● *Supporting deeper breathing*

● *Aiding balance*

Iyengar says...

❝ Remember to keep your body absolutely steady during this pose. ❞

HIGH LUNGE
Alanasana

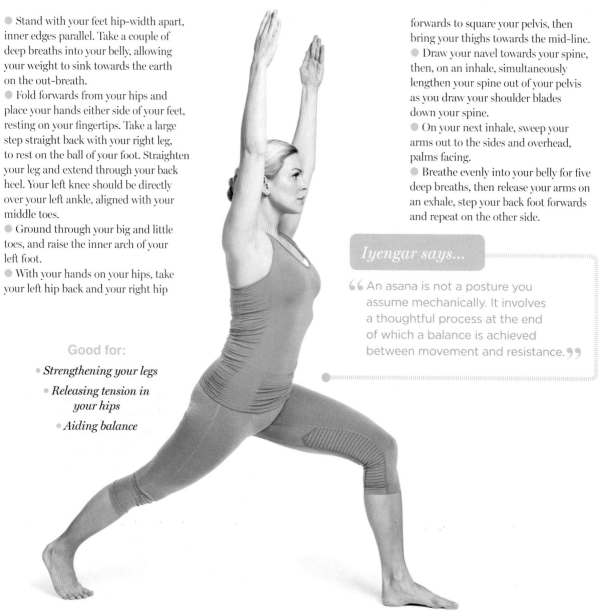

● Stand with your feet hip-width apart, inner edges parallel. Take a couple of deep breaths into your belly, allowing your weight to sink towards the earth on the out-breath.

● Fold forwards from your hips and place your hands either side of your feet, resting on your fingertips. Take a large step straight back with your right leg, to rest on the ball of your foot. Straighten your leg and extend through your back heel. Your left knee should be directly over your left ankle, aligned with your middle toes.

● Ground through your big and little toes, and raise the inner arch of your left foot.

● With your hands on your hips, take your left hip back and your right hip

forwards to square your pelvis, then bring your thighs towards the mid-line.

● Draw your navel towards your spine, then, on an inhale, simultaneously lengthen your spine out of your pelvis as you draw your shoulder blades down your spine.

● On your next inhale, sweep your arms out to the sides and overhead, palms facing.

● Breathe evenly into your belly for five deep breaths, then release your arms on an exhale, step your back foot forwards and repeat on the other side.

Iyengar says...

66 An asana is not a posture you assume mechanically. It involves a thoughtful process at the end of which a balance is achieved between movement and resistance. 99

Good for:

• *Strengthening your legs*

• *Releasing tension in your hips*

• *Aiding balance*

PYRAMID

PYRAMID
Parsvottanasana

● With your feet parallel and hip-width apart, take a large step straight back with your right leg. Keeping your left foot as it is, pivot on your right heel so your foot is at a 45-degree angle. Spread your toes and root through your left big toe and the outer edge of your right foot. Lift your inner arches by drawing your ankles apart.

● With your hands on your hips, bring your right hip forwards and your left hip back, so your pelvis is facing the front of your mat. Draw your inner thighs towards each other to stabilise the pose.

● Inhale and root down to the ground as you lengthen your spine then, on an exhale, begin to fold forwards, keeping your spine flat. Travel slowly and mindfully until you reach the end of your out-breath, then pause.

● On your next inhale, extend and lengthen your entire spine, then gently release on an exhale to fold further forwards, centring your torso over your pubis, not your front leg and letting your back naturally curve as you get lower. Continue lengthening

and lowering in this way as far as is comfortable, taking your hands to your lower legs, a block either side of your front foot if needed, or the floor.

● Rest in the pose for five to 10 breaths, breathing evenly through your nose.

When you feel ready, root through your feet and inhale to return to standing, then exhale to step your feet together. Pause for a moment, and repeat on the other side.

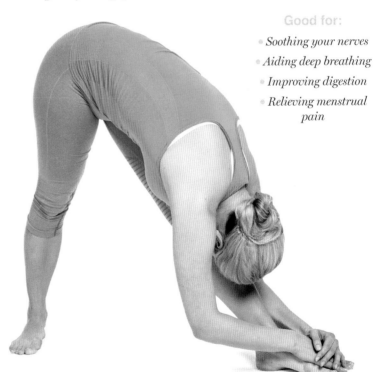

Good for:

● *Soothing your nerves*
● *Aiding deep breathing*
● *Improving digestion*
● *Relieving menstrual pain*

Iyengar says...

66 Once you become comfortable in this pose, regular practice will stimulate and tone your kidneys. It also helps remove stiffness in your neck and shoulders. 99

Vrksasana

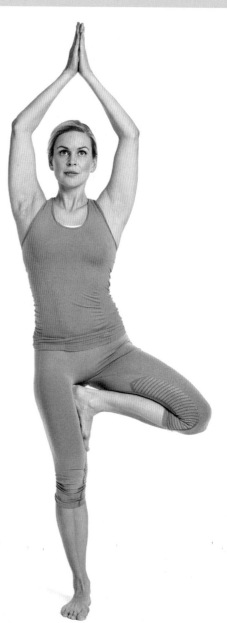

● Stand with your feet hip-distance apart and take two or three slow deep breaths to feel grounded, then transfer your weight so that it's centred over your right leg, your knee and hip stacked over your foot. Spread your toes and root through the base of your big and little toes. Lift your inner arch.

● Keeping a micro-bend in your supporting knee, focus on a fixed point ahead and grasp your left ankle, placing the sole of your left foot against your inner right thigh or calf (but not the knee area). Rest your hands on your hips.

● Keeping your hips square to the front, open your left knee out to the side, and bring your hands together in prayer position at your heart.

● Breathing slowly and deeply into your belly, press the sole of your left foot into your right thigh and engage your thigh to anchor your foot. Allow your weight to release through your right leg and foot, yielding into the ground as you feel a corresponding lift upwards through your body.

● If you feel balanced here, on your next inhale, draw your shoulder blades down

Good for:

● *Strengthening your feet, ankles, legs and core*

● *Increasing your hip and knee flexibility*

● *Aiding physical and mental balance*

● *Focusing your mind*

your back as you slowly glide your hands overhead, palms touching, elbows close to your ears.

● Finding a balance between steadiness and ease, breathe calmly in the pose as long as you feel balanced

● When you're ready, exhale and, with control, gently lower your hands and foot to return to standing. Pause for a moment with your feet together before repeating on the other side.

● As you're only in the pose a relatively short time, repeat the balance on both sides, perhaps experimenting with closed eyes if you want a stronger challenge.

Iyengar says...

" Do not forget the word align. It is through the alignment of my body I discovered the alignment of my mind, self and intelligence. "

STAFF POSE

Dandasana

● Sit with your legs straight out in front of you, feet together, ankles flexed and toes pointing to the ceiling. Rest your hands or fingertips on the floor beside your hips, fingers spread and fingertips facing forwards.

● Check that your knees are facing directly upwards and your feet are balanced on the centre of your heels. Then, when you feel ready, extend through the balls of your feet, spread your toes and reach through the base of your big and little toes. Lift your arches and draw the outside edges of your feet slightly towards your body.

● Roll your inner thighs downwards and inwards to open your sacrum, and gently shift your weight slightly forwards, to rest on the front of your sitting bones. If you find your back is curving, practise against a wall, or raise your buttocks by sitting on a low block.

● With your pelvis in neutral, root through your hands to extend out of your pelvis, draw your navel to your spine and draw your shoulder blades down your back. Lengthen the back of your neck and extend through the crown of your head.

● Breathe into your belly for 20 to 30 seconds then gently release.

Good for:

- *Focusing your mind*
- *Toning your abdominal organs*
- *Toning your back and legs*
- *Strengthening your core*

Iyengar says...

" Dandasana is the basic sitting pose for all forward bends. Practising this asana helps to increase your willpower and enhance emotional stability. "

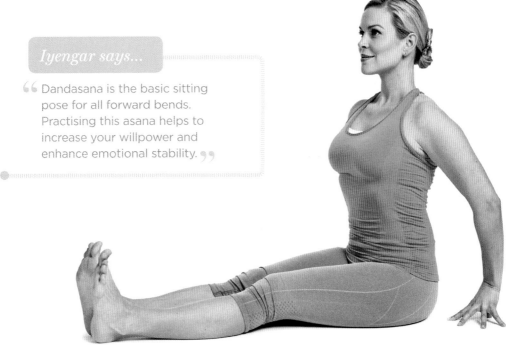

HERO POSE
Virasana

● Come onto all fours with your knees slightly apart. Have your shins parallel, tops of your feet flat on the floor and toes pointing directly backwards.

● Using your hands as a support, gently lower your sitting bones onto your heels, or, if this isn't possible, onto a block or bolster placed lengthwise between your feet. If this is uncomfortable for your ankles, place a rolled blanket beneath them before lowing your buttocks.

● Draw the flesh of your buttocks out to the sides to allow your sitting bones to separate and your tailbone to release towards the floor.

● Lift up through your spine, maintaining its vertical alignment and take your front ribs slightly in towards your back.

● Draw your shoulder blades downwards and let your head balance evenly and lightly on the top of your spine. Lengthen the back of your neck and lift up through your crown.

● Gently close your eyes and rest your hands on your thighs, palms up or down, whichever feels most comfortable.

● Breathe fully and deeply for up to one minute, gradually building up to five minutes. Let your weight sink deeper on the exhale and a gentle expansion on the inhale.

Good for:

● *Easing stiff shoulders, neck, hips, knees and groin*

● *Correcting herniated discs*

● *Relieving backache*

● *Improving circulation to your feet*

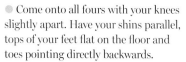

Iyengar says...

66 Virasana relieves stiffness in your joints and improves flexibility in your whole body. 99

RECLINING HERO
Supta virasana

● Place a bolster lengthwise along the centre of your mat and kneel at the bottom end. Take your knees wide as you slowly lower your buttocks onto the short end of the bolster and snuggle the inner edges of your feet against it close in to your thighs. Rest your hands on the floor either side of your hips, then root through your fingertips as you inhale and lengthen your spine. On your next exhalation, slowly lower your back onto the bolster, using your forearms to support you as you get lower.

● Rest your head on the bolster and let your arms drape alongside your body, palms facing upwards.

● Keep length in your neck by tucking in your chin, soften your throat and relax your face. Maintaining the expansion in your chest, feel the stretch from the back of your neck to your tailbone.

● Breathe deeply in the pose for up to 30 seconds, then gently engage your abdomen and press your hands into the floor to help you come up.

● Sit in an easy crossed leg pose for a few breaths.

Good for:

● *Stretching your abdomen*

● *Lengthening your thigh muscles*

● *Relieving tired legs*

● *Relieving period pains*

Iyengar says...

❝ If this pose is uncomfortable for you, raise your torso by placing a couple of blocks wrapped in a blanket underneath the head end of your bolster. ❞

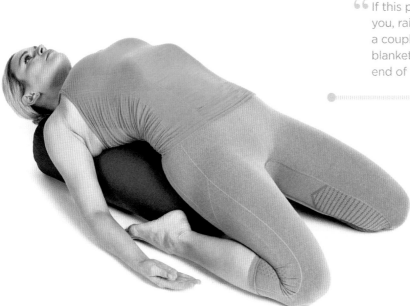

Ardha matsyendrasana

From Staff pose (p43) place your right foot outside your left knee, toes forwards and right knee pointing to the ceiling. Bend your left knee and slide your left foot to the outside of your right hip. Root down through your sitting bones. If one sitting bone comes off of the floor, or your back rounds, place a folded blanket or block beneath your raised buttock.

Wrap your left arm around your right knee and rest your right fingertips on the floor behind you (pictured). If comfortable, inhale to raise your left hand, and on an exhale, take your elbow outside your left knee, forearm vertical and palm facing the right. Keep your spine vertical and draw your shoulder blades into your back.

Good for:

- *Easing tension in your back*
- *Toning your spinal nerves*
- *Opening your chest*
- *Relieving stiff hips*

Inhale as you root through your fingers and sitting bones to lengthen your spine, then as you exhale, twist to the right. Move a little deeper into the stretch with each breath, lengthening your spine on the inhale, releasing a little deeper into the twist on the exhale.

Turn your head to gaze over your right shoulder, breathing evenly from your belly for another five breaths.

Inhale to move back to centre, then pause before repeating on the other side.

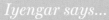

Iyengar says...

66 In twists, your spine becomes more supple, and this improves the flow of blood to your spinal nerves and increases energy levels. 99

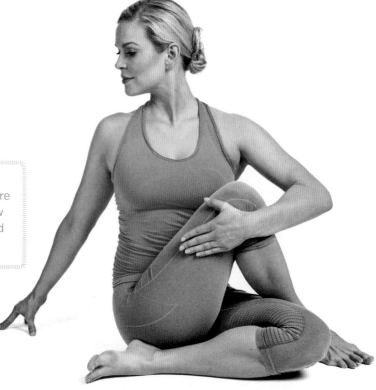

RELAXATION
Savasana

● Lie on your back and extend your arms a comfortable distance from your sides, palms facing upwards. Extend your legs, taking your feet a little wider than hip-distance apart, and allow your feet to roll out to the sides.

● Wriggle your torso a little, to snuggle your body into the floor then, checking that your arms and legs are symmetrical, rest your head on the centre of the back of your skull. Gently close your eyes.

● Allow any tension built up in your practice to release into the floor, consciously letting go on each exhalation.

● Breathe softly and evenly into your belly, letting your eyelids be heavy, your jaw soft and your belly relaxed.

Rest for a few moments, then let your breath become a little slower and deeper, making your out-breath slightly longer than your in-breath. Allow any tension to sink into the mat as you breathe out.

● Spend some time reflecting on the pose you have focused on today, notice any changes in your body after having worked in the pose. What feels stretched? What felt challenging?

● Let your breath return to normal, and rest in the pose for five to 10 minutes. Notice if you can feel a gentle sense of expansion as you inhale, and a feeling of softening as you exhale.

● To come out of the pose, slowly wriggle your fingers and toes. Slide your arms out to the sides and overhead, and gently stretch your body from your feet to your fingertips. Slowly bring your knees to your chest, roll over to your right-hand side and rest for few moments, then use your left hand to help you come up to sitting.

Good for:

● *Calming your mind*

● *Balancing your mind, body and spirit*

● *Rejuvenating*

● *Reducing fatigue*

Iyengar says...

66 In Savasana, your body and mind become one, and you experience inner silence. 99

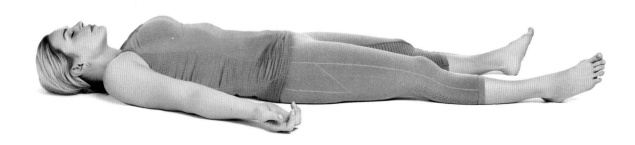

THE IYENGAR
sequence

*Improve your **alignment***

This session invites you to commit to focusing on your form. Take your time studying the alignment guides on the preceding pages and spend the first few moments in the pose scanning your body to check you are well balanced and following the suggested guidelines. When you are confident of your form, release the mental connection and let your attention return to your breath, allowing yourself to sink more deeply into the pose. Ujjayi breathing will help you focus and turn inwards.

When you feel ready, take a final deep breath and mindfully come out of the pose. You might light to pause for a moment or two (in Mountain pose, p36, for the standing section or Hero, p44, for the seated section) to register the effects of the pose before moving on to the next.

The moves

START

Warm-up
Choose one or two moves from each section of the spine, hip and shoulder sections in the warm-ups on pages 20–23.

Pranayama
Ujjayi (p35)
Sun salute
Sun salute II (p26)

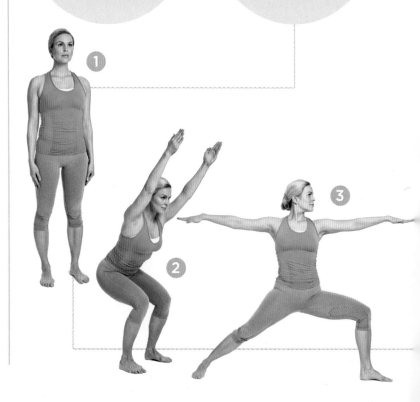

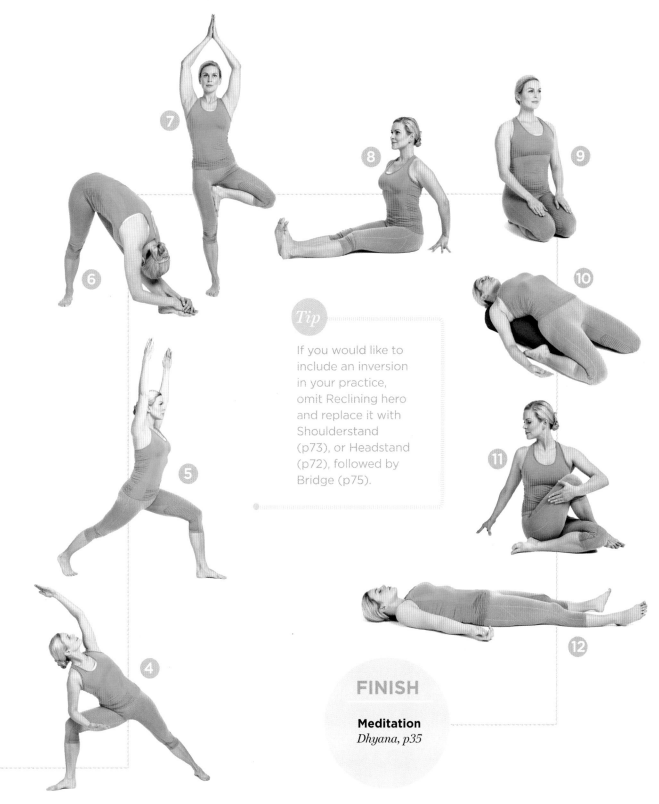

Tip

If you would like to include an inversion in your practice, omit Reclining hero and replace it with Shoulderstand (p73), or Headstand (p72), followed by Bridge (p75).

FINISH

Meditation
Dhyana, p35

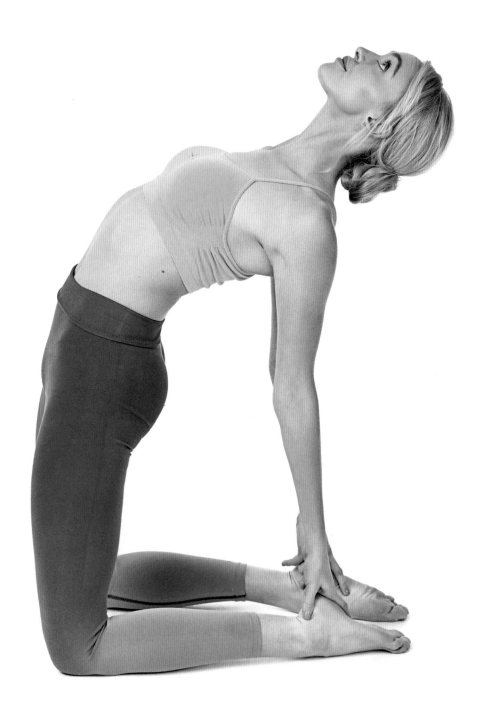

Vinyasa

Now you've become familiar with the **alignment** principles of some key yoga poses, it's time to get a feel for a style of yoga that joins asanas together in one continuous flow. Vinyasa, a **sanskrit** word that means 'to place in a special way', seamlessly combines postures to create a fluid movement practice – in the way that **t'ai chi** does. Sometimes described as consciousness in motion, Vinyasa is a good choice to make when you want to develop a more **mindful way** of being to help you stay connected to your inner self when you're faced with the multifaceted aspects of life. Depending on the postures chosen for a sequence, the speed at which you practise and the number of **repetitions** you include, a Vinyasa session can feel like a calming meditative flow or an energising cardio workout.

INTRODUCTION TO
Vinyasa

Vinyasa yoga is a generic term for many varied yoga styles, such as Power Flow, Vinyasa Flow and the soft, fluid moves of Shiva Rea's Prana Vinyasa, but its origins can be traced back to Ashtanga, created by Sri K Pattabhi Jois in 1948, who, along with Iyengar was a student of Sri Krishnamacharya in India, and one of the founding fathers of modern yoga. Ashtanga involves a series of around 50 postures performed in order in six separate 'series'. It's a demanding, sweaty, energising practice with classes sometimes lasting two hours, that can help you shape up, lose weight and build stamina. It's also believed to purify the body and rejuvenate the mind, and strict Astangis will also adhere to spiritual practices that include following certain moral codes.

The Vinyasa we are sharing with you here is a gentle introduction to the form, and one that encourages you to be aware of your body moment to moment as you move through the form. Pay as much attention to the transitions as to the poses themselves – staying present throughout your practice is central to Vinyasa.

> **"** *We're sharing a gentle introduction to Vinyasa that encourages you to be more aware of your body moment to moment* **"**

BEFORE YOU BEGIN

● As well as describing a particular yoga style, Vinyasa is often used to describe a short sequence of linked poses: Plank, Four-limbed staff pose (or Caterpillar), Upward dog (or Cobra) and Downward dog. In a class when a teacher says, 'take a Vinyasa' this is likely what they are referring to. We'll include a few of these mini Vinyasas in our sequence, using Caterpillar and Cobra to make the sequence suitable for beginners. If you've been practising Vinyasa for a while, feel free to substitute these suggestions for Four-limbed staff pose and Upward dog.

● To help you stay present and connected to the flowing style of this sequence, remember to stay connected to your breath. You might also like to play a soft, flowing piece of music to help you tune in to a meditative space.

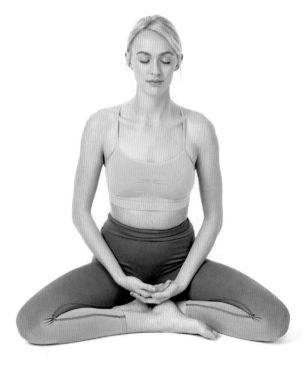

Pranayama

SVARA PRANAYAMA
Yoga of sound breath

▦ In yoga philosophy, different parts of your nostril linings are associated with the five elements: water, fire, air, earth and 'ether'. And by channelling your breath as you inhale, it is believed that you can influence the expression of these qualities in your mind and body.

▦ This preparatory technique for the full svara pranayama helps you become more aware of your breath and gain greater control over it. Sitting in a comfortable position, spend some time breathing into your abdomen to help you let go of the day. When you feel centred, return to normal breathing and bring your attention to your nostrils. Become aware of the sensations in your nose as you breathe in – does the air feel cool or warm? – and as you breathe out – is it the same temperature? Spend a few moments here, then notice if you can feel where the air touches the surface of your nostrils as it passes by – can you feel it grazing your inner nostril, by the septum?

▦ Do you notice any sensation on your outer nostril, beneath the 'wing' of your nose? Continue refining your experience of your breath for a few more moments, then try narrowing your nostrils. What to you notice now? After a couple of minutes, 'flare' your nostrils, making them spread wide. Does your breath feel different now? If it helps, as you inhale, try raising your arms to your side to shoulder height or above. Spend two minutes here then return to normal breathing for a few moments, and gently open your eyes.

Meditation

SACRAL CHAKRA MEDITATION

▦ Flow is connected with the element water, and water is associated with the sacral chakra, also known as the hara, which is located two fingers'-width below your navel. To begin, sit in a comfortable position and take your attention to the area around your hara, noticing any sensations you feel – heat, fullness, tingling or maybe nothing at all. Observe without judgement. Now, as you breathe in, imagine you are breathing in through a nostril situated at your hara. Take a long slow inhalation through your hara, then imagine your breath slowly leaving your body by the hara as you exhale.

▦ Continue breathing in this way for about five minutes, gradually letting your mind become still as you allow your sensitivity to remain open. When you've finished, place your palms over your navel, one on top of the other and hold your belly for a few moments to ground your experience.

Utthita balasana

Kneeling on your mat, take three breaths into your belly, then draw your knees apart and bring your big toes together, heels wide. Sit back on the soles of your feet and rest your palms on your thighs.

Inhale as you root into your sitting bones to lengthen your spine. On an exhale, slowly walk your hands forwards, as you lower your torso between your thighs.

Take your hands shoulder-width apart, palms down, fingers spread and middle finger pointing forwards. Actively root your hands into the floor, keep your elbows off the mat and draw your arms into your arm sockets as you slide your shoulder blades down your back.

Exhale and lower your head, gently resting your forehead on the floor, a block or a bolster, depending on your flexibility. Softly close your eyes.

Breathe deeply and evenly into your back body for five breaths, sinking deeper into the mat on each exhale. As you extend through to your fingertips, reach your tailbone back to your heels.

On an exhale, use your hands to gently bring you up to a comfortable seated position. Pause a moment to register the effects of the pose.

Good for:
- *Opening your groin*
- *Relieving stress and fatigue*
- *Nurturing*
- *Calming your mind*

Tip

To help you fold from your hips rather than waist, place your thumbs in your hip creases (between the top of your thighs and lower abdomen) and push down and backwards before folding forwards.

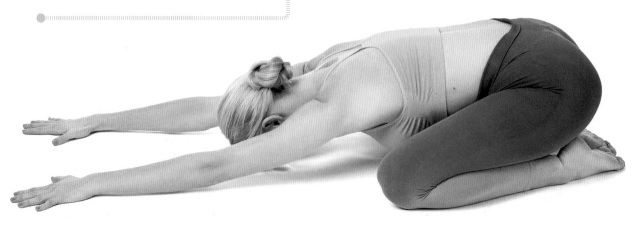

EASY POSE

Sukhasana

Sit on your mat and cross your legs at your shins, so your lower legs are parallel to the front edge of your mat. Use your hands to draw one buttock then the other away from your mid-line to help you root into the ground through your sitting bones.

Flex your feet to stabilise and protect your knees, then place your hands (or fingertips) either side of your hips, and root down as you draw your navel to your spine and lengthen up out of your pelvis.

Open your chest, draw your shoulder blades down your back and lift through your crown. Lengthen the back of your neck and softly close your eyes, or gaze a few feet in front of you on the floor.

Rest your hands on your thighs, palms facing upwards, and allow your weight to sink into the floor on each exhale. Let your mind become still.

Breathe calmly and evenly into your abdomen as long as is comfortable, then gently open your eyes.

Good for:

- *Grounding and centring*
- *Soothing your nervous system*
- *Calming and settling your mind*

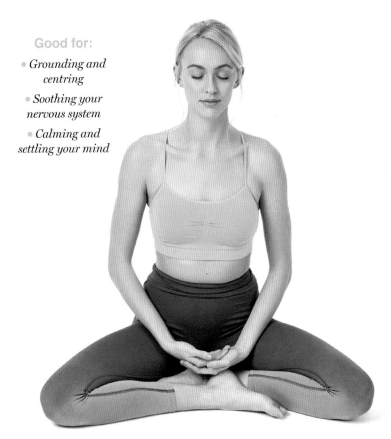

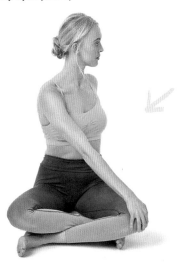

VARIATION
Easy twist

From easy pose, place your left hand on the floor behind your left buttock, fingers pointing backwards, and rest your right palm on the outside of your left knee. Inhale as you root through your sitting bones to lift your spine out of your pelvis. On an exhale, slowly rotate your spine to the left, moving in a spiral from your waist initially, then your upper body. Inhale, lengthen through the crown of your head, exhale further into the twist. Draw the kidney area forwards and abdomen towards your navel. Inhale one last time, exhale, release further into the twist, turning your head to look over your left shoulder if comfortable for your neck. Inhale back to centre and repeat on the other side.

CRESCENT
Anjaneyasana

● From standing, fold forwards and place your hands either side of your feet. Slide your left leg back and lower onto your knee and the top of your foot. Adjust your right foot, if needed, so your knee is over your ankle. Spread your right toes and lift your inner arch.

● Inhale and raise your torso to vertical, tucking under your tailbone, squaring your hips and drawing your navel towards your spine. As you exhale, sink into your hips.

● Interlace your fingers and thumbs, index fingers pointing forwards, and inhale as you bring your arms forwards and over your head.

● Take five to 10 deep breaths into your belly, then lower your hands and place either side of your front foot. Step forwards with your back foot and slowly uncurl your spine to return to standing. Repeat on the other side.

Good for:

- *Balancing*
- *Gently energising*
- *Strengthening your legs*
- *Opening your hip flexors*

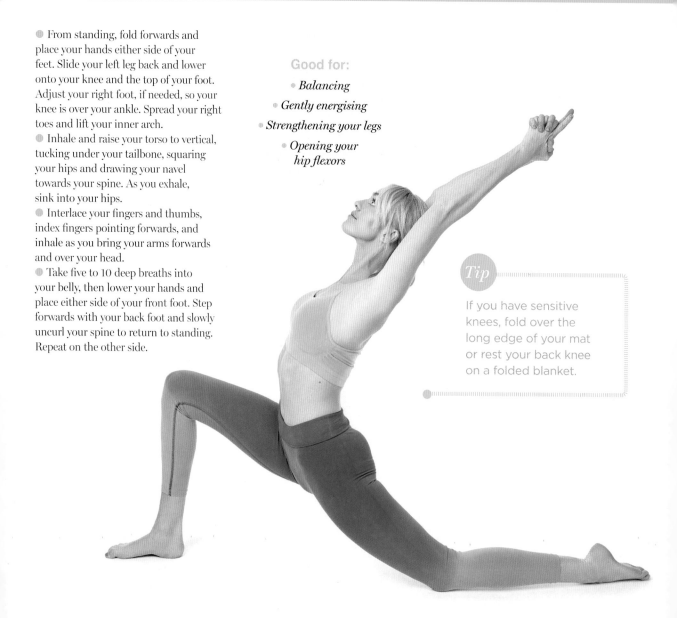

Tip

If you have sensitive knees, fold over the long edge of your mat or rest your back knee on a folded blanket.

DOWNWARD DOG SPLITS
Eka pada adho mukha svanasana

● From Downward dog (p110), step your feet together then, inhale as you sweep your right leg back and up, lifting from your hip. Draw your right hip forwards and your left hip back to keep your pelvis square, and internally rotate your raised leg, so your knee and the top of your foot point down towards the mat.

● Root through the base of your thumbs and index fingers, and externally rotate your upper arms. Draw your shoulder blades away from each other and down your spine to create space around your neck.

● Continue lengthening your spine evenly through both sides of your waist and extend your right leg further, to create a straight line from your crown right through to your raised foot.

● After five deep breaths, exhale as you lower your leg. Pause for a moment, then repeat on the other side.

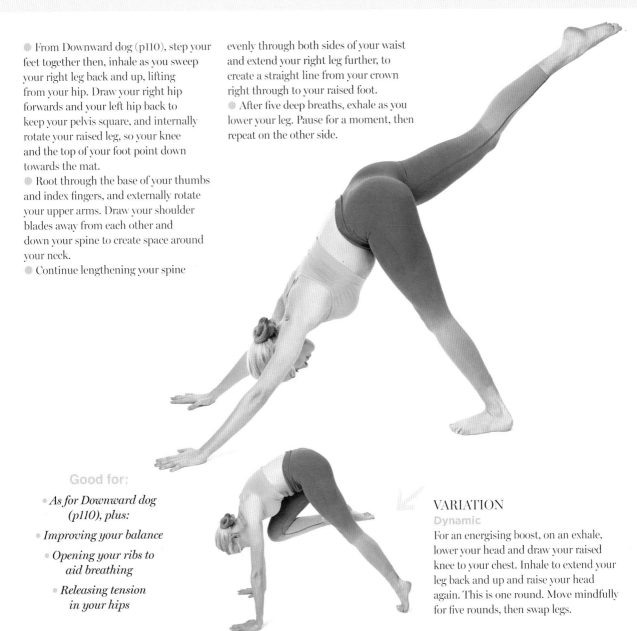

Good for:

● *As for Downward dog (p110), plus:*

● *Improving your balance*

● *Opening your ribs to aid breathing*

● *Releasing tension in your hips*

VARIATION
Dynamic

For an energising boost, on an exhale, lower your head and draw your raised knee to your chest. Inhale to extend your leg back and up and raise your head again. This is one round. Move mindfully for five rounds, then swap legs.

Kumbhakasana

Start on all fours with your hands shoulder-width apart, directly beneath your shoulders. Spread your fingers, root through the base of your thumb and index finger and straighten your elbows without locking them.

Step your feet back, resting on the balls of your feet, and straighten your legs to create a diagonal line from your heels to your crown. Tuck in your chin to maintain length in the back of your neck.

Draw your navel to your spine and spread your shoulder blades apart.

Breathe evenly for five to 10 breaths, then gently lower on an exhale.

Tip

Reach your heels to the back of your mat and extend to the crown of your head. Beginners, start on your knees and tops of your toes and build your strength gradually.

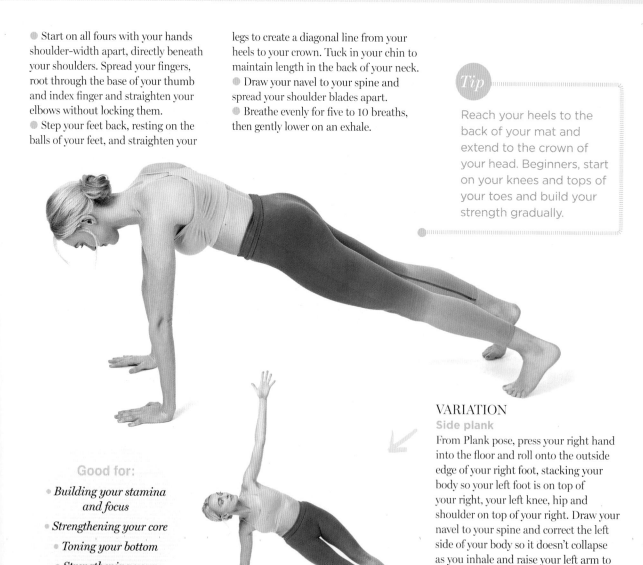

Good for:

- *Building your stamina and focus*
- *Strengthening your core*
- *Toning your bottom*
- *Strengthening your upper body*

VARIATION
Side plank

From Plank pose, press your right hand into the floor and roll onto the outside edge of your right foot, stacking your body so your left foot is on top of your right, your left knee, hip and shoulder on top of your right. Draw your navel to your spine and correct the left side of your body so it doesn't collapse as you inhale and raise your left arm to the ceiling. If you need to, bend your top knee and rest your foot behind the knee of your straight leg.

HALF MOON
Ardha chandrasana

From Triangle (p83), step your right foot in slightly and place your right hand on a block about a foot in front and slightly outside your right foot.

Keeping your right leg bent, place your left hand on your left hip and root through your right foot as you lean into the block until your left leg feels 'empty'. Inhale as you float your left leg up to hip height. Flex your rear ankle, spread your toes and extend through the ball of your left foot.

Ground your right foot into the floor as you straighten your supporting leg and rotate your chest and pelvis open to the left, so your hips and shoulders are stacked one above the other.

Keeping a soft gaze towards the floor, inhale and raise your left hand up to the ceiling.

Breathe evenly from your belly for three to five breaths, imagining there are lines of energy travelling from your centre out through each limb.

Once you can balance well using the block, place your hand on the floor instead, remembering to spread your fingertips and root into the ground to lift your torso upwards.

Exhale to lower, then pause in Wide-legged forward fold (p116) before repeating on the other side.

Good for:
- *Aiding balance and focus*
- *Helping to relieve stress and anxiety*
- *Easing fatigue*
- *Opening your ribs/ improving breathing*

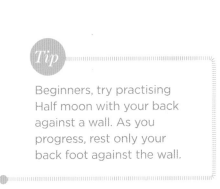

Tip

Beginners, try practising Half moon with your back against a wall. As you progress, rest only your back foot against the wall.

CAMEL
Ustrasana

- Kneel on a mat with your thighs hip-width apart, the front of your toes resting on the mat.
- Inhale, lengthen your spine and circle your left arm over your head and rest it on your left ankle, fingers pointing to your buttocks. Exhale.
- On your next inhale, repeat the same move with your right hand, eyes looking ahead so you don't strain your neck. Exhale.
- As you inhale, lift your sternum gently upwards, opening your chest and shoulders. Release your tailbone to the floor to feel the stretch in your quads and core.
- Maintain the length in your neck, and tuck your chin in slightly.
- Take five to 10 deep breaths, then release on an exhale and rest in Child's pose.

Good for:

- *Boosting your energy*
- *Opening your chest and heart*
- *Strengthening your thighs*
- *Opening your hip flexors*

Tip

If you are new to Camel, practise the pose with your toes turned under and rest your hands on blocks on the outside of your ankles.

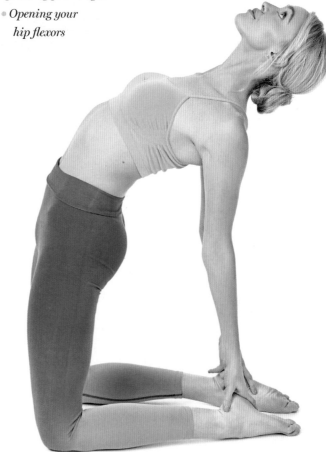

BOAT

Navasana

● Sit on your mat, bend your knees, raise your feet off the floor and grasp the back of your thighs with your hands.

● Draw your navel to your spine and lean back to balance on your sitting bones. Take a few breaths here, then raise your lower legs until your shins are parallel to the floor.

● If you're comfortable here, extend your arms and hold them parallel to the floor. Take another few breaths and raise your arms and, if you feel balanced, straighten your legs to take your body into a 'V' shape.

● Draw your shoulder blades down your spine and keep your abdominals engaged but your feet relaxed. Take up to five breaths before releasing on an exhale.

Good for:

- *Aiding focus*
- *Easing stress*
- *Toning your abdominals*
- *Strengthening your back muscles*

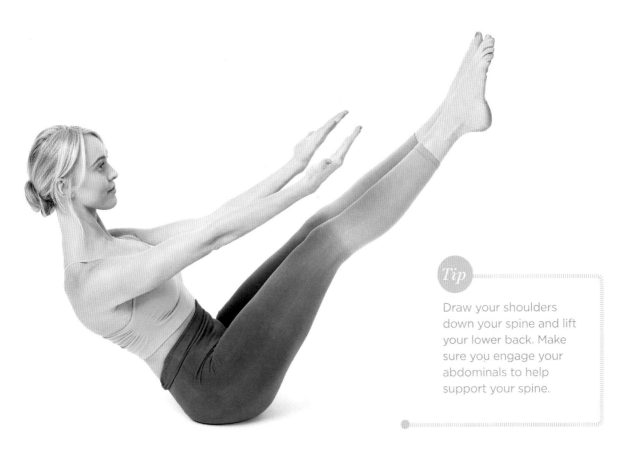

Tip

Draw your shoulders down your spine and lift your lower back. Make sure you engage your abdominals to help support your spine.

WHEEL
Urdhva dhanurasana

● Lie on your back, knees bent and heels close to your buttocks. Place your palms on the floor beside your shoulders, fingertips pointing to your feet, elbows in and pointing upwards.

● On an inhale, press your hands and feet into the floor and raise your hips up and back. Raise your head and rest your crown on the floor. Check your elbows are shoulder-width-apart. Exhale.

● On your next inhale, press into the floor and straighten your arms and legs to lift your body.

● Release your neck and imagine your body being lifted up by your navel. Take five deep breaths, then lower with control on an exhale by gently bending your arms and legs, taking care of your neck by placing the back of your head on your mat.

Good for:

- *Boosting energy*
- *Soothing stress*
- *Strengthening your thighs, shoulders, arms, wrists and spine*

Tip

If you're new to this pose, make sure you're proficient at Bridge (p75), then build up to Wheel by placing two blocks against a wall and alternate resting your hands or your feet on them, to lessen the depth of the backbend.

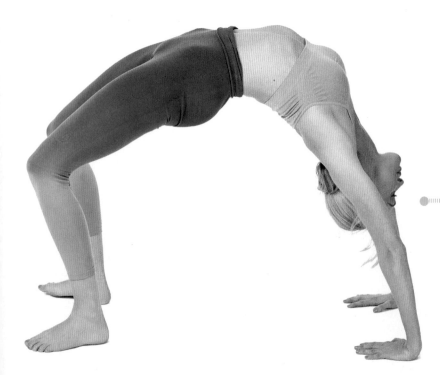

RECLINING TWIST

RECLINING TWIST
Supta parivartanasana

● Lie on your back and take a few moments to centre yourself, allowing your breath to deepen and your heartbeat to become slower.

● Hug both knees to your chest, using your forearms to bring your knees in close and draw your shoulder blades down your back. Take a few breaths here, then extend your right leg to the floor, allowing your right thigh to release down to the mat.

● Rest your right hand on your left knee and on an exhale, guide it over to the right. Extend your left arm to the side and, if comfortable, gently turn your head to look to the left.

● Breathe deeply into your left side, enjoying the stretch for 10 deep breaths, then slowly inhale back to centre and repeat on the other side.

Good for:

● *Reducing stress*
● *Releasing tension in your spine*
● *Opening your chest*
● *Easing stiffness in your lower back*

Tip

To facilitate this twist and maintain good alignment of your spine, before you begin, lift your buttocks and shift them slightly to the left before twisting to the right, and vice versa.

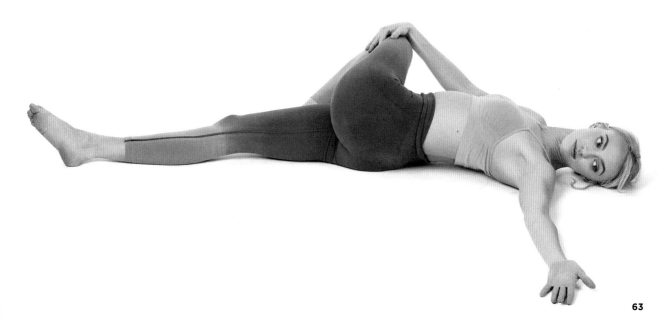

THE VINYASA
sequence

Calm and energise

This sequence follows a traditional yoga class, beginning with standing poses, moving on to seated postures and an inversion (your head is lower than your heart). Choose a Sun Salute according to your energy levels and, for a challenge, include a mini Vinyasa (p65) each time you come into Downward dog (p110). While you're learning the poses, pause for a few breaths in each one to refine your alignment. When you're more familiar with the moves, use the breathing pattern below, remaining fully present in the transitions between poses. Move slowly and mindfully for a calming flow, or work faster for an energising boost.

The moves

START

Warm-up
Choose one or two moves from each section of the spine, hip and shoulder sections in the warm-ups on pages 20-23.

Pranayama
Yoga of sound breath (p53)

Sun salute
Sun salute I (p24) or Sun salute II (p26)

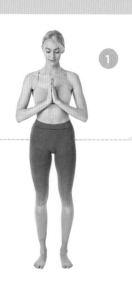

1

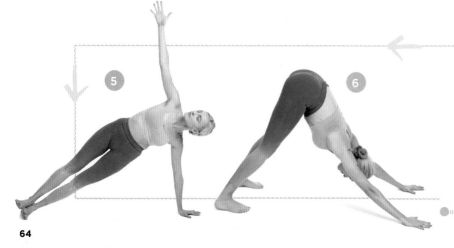

5

6

Tip

Land as lightly as you can when stepping your back foot between your hands from Downward dog.

1 Mountain (p36)
Inhale and reach your arms out to the sides and overhead into...

2 Extended mountain (p36)
Exhale as you take your arms out to the side and fold with a flat back into...

3 Standing forward fold (p82)
Inhale and step both feet back into...

4 Plank (p58)

Rest here for 5 breaths then inhale and lift your right arm to come into...

5 Side plank (p58)
Rest here for five breaths then exhale, lower your hand back into Plank and swap sides, raising your left arm on an inhalation. Return to Plank on an exhalation then step both feet back into...

6 Downward dog (p110)
Rest for a moment or

do a mini Vinyasa, then raise your left leg to come into...

7 Downward dog splits x3 (p57)
Step your left raised leg forwards between your hands to come into...

8 Crescent (p56)
Lower both hands to the floor, then inhale and cartwheel your left arm forwards, overhead and back as you come into...

Mini Vinyasa

Every time the guidelines invite you to do a mini Vinyasa, do the following poses in one continuous flow. If you're feeling energetic, repeat the mini Vinyasa once or twice more before continuing with the main sequence.

1 Downward dog
Exhale into...
2 Plank Pause the breath as you lower into...
3 Caterpillar Inhale as you lift into...
4 Cobra Inhale, then exhale into...
5 Downward dog

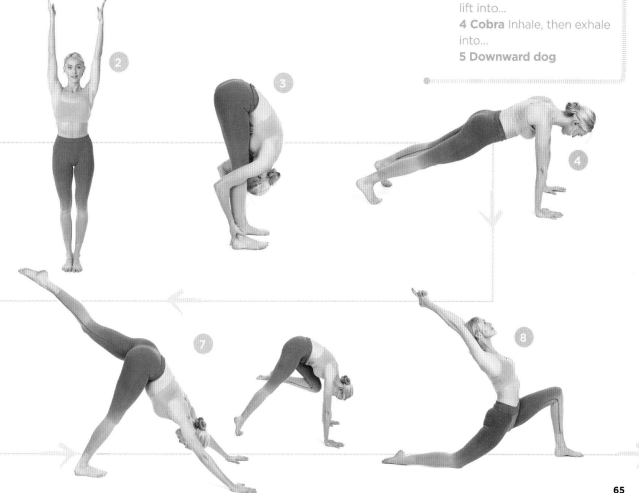

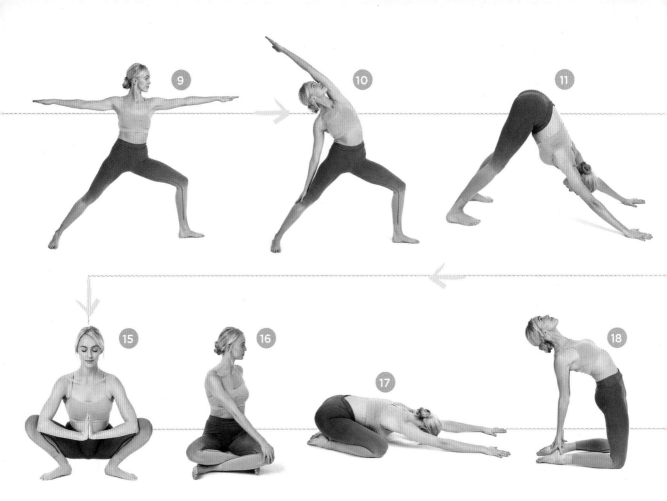

9 Warrior II (p38)
On an inhale, circle your left arm overhead and slide your right arm down your back thigh to come into...

10 Reverse warrior x3 (p38)
Repeat 9 and 10 three times, exhaling into Warrior II and inhaling into Reverse warrior. Then from Warrior II inhale and exhale as you cartwheel your left arm overhead and down to your mat to come into...

11 Downward dog (p110)
Rest here for a moment

or do a mini Vinyasa. Then repeat 7-10 on the other leg. Inhale to raise your left leg into Downward dog splits (7), then exhale as you step your left foot between your hands. Inhale to come up into ...

12 Triangle (p83)
Place your left hand about a foot in front of your left foot and slightly to the outside. Step your back foot a little closer to your front foot, then raise your right leg to come into...

13 Half moon (p59)
Exhale to lower your right arm and leg then pivot on your feet to face the side of your mat, and walk your hands between your legs into....

14 Wide-legged forward fold (p116)
Walk your hands back to the front of your mat and step back into Downward dog (11), taking a rest or doing a mini Vinyasa. Repeat 4-14 on the other side then walk your hands back to your feet, bend your knees and lower into...

15 Garland (p81)
Lower onto your buttocks and sit cross-legged for five breaths, then place your right hand on your left knee, and your left hand behind you to come into...

16 Easy twist (p54)
Repeat on the other side, then come onto your knees, big toes touching, knees spread and walk your hands forwards into...

17 Extended child's pose (p55)
Rest for five breaths.

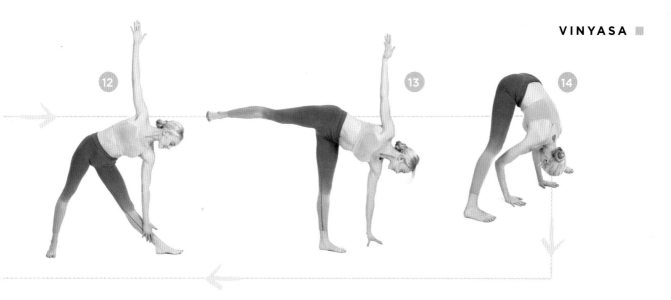

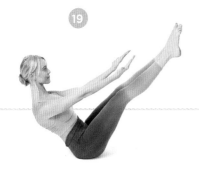

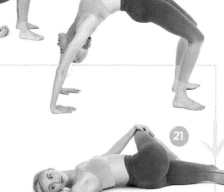

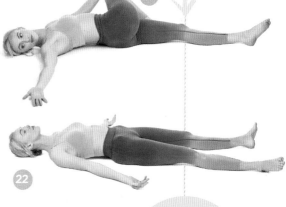

Walk your hands to the right and the left, then back to centre and come to kneeling, to move into...

18 Camel (p60)
Lower onto all fours, then keeping your knees where they are, swing your feet out to the side and lower your buttocks onto to the opposite side of your hips. Exhale as you raise your arms and legs into...

19 Boat (p61)
Slowly lower your arms and legs on an exhale, rest a moment, and

then, depending on your experience, inhale into...

20 Bridge or Wheel (p75) or (p62)
Exhale as you lower your body to your mat with control. Rest a moment then come into...

21 Reclining twist (p63)
Rest for five breaths. Repeat on the other side, then centre your body on your mat and relax back into...

22 Savasana (p47)
Rest here for seven to 10 minutes.

FINISH

Meditation
Sacral chakra (p53)

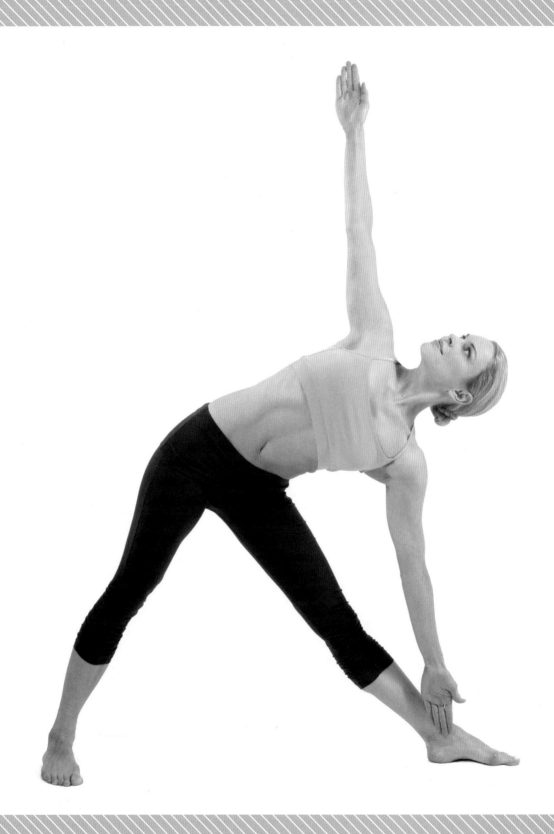

Sivananda

Congratulations on reaching the **halfway point** in your yoga exploration. By now you'll be familiar with many of the **principles of asana**, have learnt some valuable breathing and meditation techniques and started to enjoy the benefits of regular practice. If you feel you've been taking in a lot of new information, and want to hone in on just a few poses, Sivananda could be the ideal style for you. Work with this chapter whenever you want to experience more **serenity in your life**. Our sequence follows the same format you'll see in a Sivananda class – 12 specific poses practised in the same order each session – and is a great option to choose when you want a more **structured approach** to learning and where you can observe your improvements week on week.

INTRODUCTION TO
Sivananda

Swami Sivananda was originally a medical doctor, but after curing a wandering monk who taught him asana and yogic philosophy, he began a 10-year spiritual journey, that led ultimately to the foundation of Sivananda yoga. It was brought to the West in the 1950s by a disciple of his, Swami Vishnudevananda, who went on to write the authoritative guide to the style, *The Complete Illustrated Book of Yoga* (Crown, £15.99).

Perhaps best summed up by the words Serve, Love, Give, Purify, Meditate and Realise, Sivananda yoga believes that the path to physical health, mental wellbeing and spiritual growth is achieved through proper exercise, proper breathing, proper relaxation, proper diet, positive thinking and meditation. Yoga asanas, pranayama, a lacto-vegetarian diet (simple, natural ingredients following ayurvedic principles) and a meditative spiritual practice paves the way for vibrant health and a peaceful, joyful mind.

'When the surface of a lake is still, one can see to the bottom very clearly. This is impossible when the surface is agitated by waves. In the same way, when the mind is still, with no thoughts or desires, you can see the "Self" this is called Yoga.' *International Yoga Vendanta Centre*

> 66 *Sivananda yoga is best summed up by the words Serve, Love, Give, Purify, Meditate and Realise* 99

BEFORE YOU BEGIN

● Traditionally, Sivananda classes begin with leg lifts as a warm-up, so we begin our session with Single and Double leg lifts. If, after trying them before the sequence on p84, you feel you need a longer warm-up, chose one or two moves from each of the spine, shoulder and hip warm-ups on page 20-23.

● Single leg lifts: lie on your back with your arms at your sides, palms facing down, legs straight and ankles flexed. Slowly inhale as you raise your right leg to a count of five, taking it as high as you comfortably can without bending your knee. On an exhale, lower to a count of five, then raise your left leg. Repeat five to 10 times.

● Double leg lifts: as before, only this time, raise both legs together, keeping them straight. Aim to bring your legs to vertical if possible, repeating five to eight times.

● Breathe deeply and evenly into your abdomen throughout the session, or you may want to use Ujjayi breathing (p35).

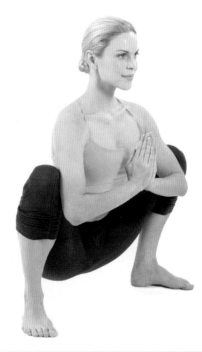

Pranayama

KAPALABHATI

■ Also known as the cleansing breath or skull shining breath, this exercise energises your whole body very quickly. Do not practise it if you are pregnant, menstruating or after eating. Sit in a comfortable position and connect to your breathing for a few moments to centre yourself. When you're ready, place your hands on your belly and draw your navel in and up as you exhale quickly through your nose. Rather than consciously breathing in, allow inhalation to happen naturally. Repeat this four to eight times, noticing your belly move in and out like a bellows beneath your hands. End with an out-breath.

■ This is one cycle. Do three or four more, increasing the speed of your breath, so each exhalation lasts one second. Take a few, deep Ujjayi breaths (p35) after each cycle to rest your lungs and diaphragm. You can build up to 15–30 breaths per cycle.

Sound meditation

■ If you have difficulty visualising things, you could meditate on a sound, such as a ticking clock or birdsong. Spend a few moments arriving in your body, then close your eyes and give your attention to your chosen sound. Try not to extend your energy out to the sound to hear it, but let the sound to come to you – simply 'receive' the sound. If there are many sounds around you, choose the one you're drawn to and hone in on it.

■ Enjoy the sense of stillness you get by attuning yourself to one thing. If you're listening to an intermittent sound, such as birdsong, sink into the silence between the sounds. Gently open your eyes to finish, maintaining the sense of equilibrium.

Meditation

TRATAK

■ We begin with an exercise that helps you cultivate concentration. Spend a few moments calming your thoughts and becoming present – closing your eyes and directing your attention to your breath. Then, when you feel centred, open your eyes and, without blinking, focus on an object, such as a candle or a single point in front of you. Once you blink, close your eyes and visualise this object in your mind's eye and concentrate on the mental image. Many people say they find it difficult to 'empty their mind', but regular practice of this will help quieten racing thoughts by teaching you to focus on one thing only. Each time you return to the exercise, use the same object. Ultimately, this exercise can lead towards one-pointed concentration.

Flower meditation

■ Try this practice if you're a visual person. Get into a comfortable sitting position and spend a few moments to become centred, then draw your attention inwards. When you feel ready, close your eyes and spend a few moments imagining that you're walking through a beautiful garden in early summer. You are surrounded by flowers, gently swaying in the soft warm breeze.

■ After a while, gradually allow yourself to be drawn to one particular flower and begin to focus your attention on it. Become absorbed by its colour, shape, texture and allow the fragrance to permeate you. Stay connected to your experience as long as possible. When you finish, take a couple of deep breaths then gently open your eyes.

Salamba sirsasana

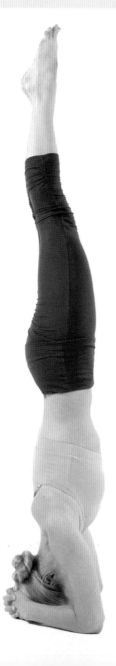

● Begin on all-fours and lower your forearms to the floor, elbows shoulder-distance apart. Clasp your hands together with your fingers interlaced and thumbs resting on your index fingers and rest your hands on your little finger edge.
● Lean forwards and rest the front of the crown of your head on the floor then cup your head with your hands. Keep your neck long and your shoulders away from your ears. Straighten your legs, lifting your buttocks and rest on the tips of your toes. Slowly edge your toes forwards as far as you can while keeping your legs straight.
● When your hips are over your shoulders, engage your core, bend your knees and lift them to your chest so you are in a reverse tuck position, torso vertical, knees pointing down and toes pointing to the ceiling. Keep contracting your core as you slowly extend your legs straight upwards, ankles flexed.
● Keep rooting through your forearms and wrists then lift strongly through your inner and outer legs. Breathe steadily.
● Remain in the pose for 10 to 20 breaths, gradually increasing the time to 10 minutes.
● To come down, on an exhale, slowly and with control, come out of the pose in the way you went in - lowering into a reverse tuck, then walking your feet away from your head. Rest for a moment in Relaxation pose (p47).

Good for:

- *Calming your mind*
- *Increasing your concentration*
- *Improving your circulation*
- *Strengthening your shoulders, arms and core*

Sivananda benefit

The king of asanas relaxes and enlivens your entire body.

SHOULDERSTAND

Salamba sarvangasana

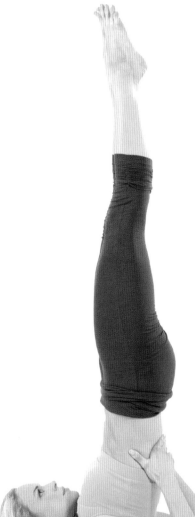

● Lie on your back with your knees bent, feet flat on the floor and arms at your sides.

● Bring your knees over your chest then exhale and root through your elbows to lift your buttocks to the ceiling and your knees towards your head. Rest your hands on your back to support your spine.

● Draw your shoulder blades together and bring your elbows close to your body. On an exhale, take your hips over your shoulders and slowly raise your feet towards the ceiling. Reach up strongly, lengthening your inner and outer legs upwards, so your body is perpendicular to the floor from your shoulders to your toes.

● Draw your shoulder blades down your spine and in towards your heart and lift your sternum to vertical.

● Draw the sides of your waist horizontally towards your centre, and your upper and lower abdomen vertically towards your navel. This will support your spine and help

maintain the lift in your torso and legs.

● Remain in the pose for 10 to 20 breaths gradually increasing the time to five minutes, breathing slowly and evenly into your belly.

● To come out, bend your knees in to your chest, release your arms and on an exhale, slowly uncurl your spine to release down to the floor, one vertebra at a time. Rest in Relaxation pose (p47).

Good for:

● *Helping tiredness and stress*

● *Stimulating your thyroid gland*

● *Stretching your shoulders and back*

● *Aiding insomnia*

Sivananda benefit

The queen of yoga poses, Shoulderstand opens your neck and upper back.

SUPPORTED PLOUGH
Halasana

Lie on your back with your arms by your sides, palms down. As you exhale, push your hands into the mat, draw your navel to your spine to contract your abdominals and bring your knees to your chest, curling your body into a ball.

Using this momentum, swing your feet over your head as you take your hands to your hips to support your lower back. Continue rolling back, allowing your toes to rest on the floor behind you.

For now, slightly round your torso and keep your knees bent. Keep your gaze towards your thighs, as this will protect your neck from any damage.

As you become acclimatised to the pose, lift your hips to bring them directly above your shoulders, draw your hands down your spine to support your upper back and begin to extend your heels away to gradually straighten your legs.

If you feel comfortable here, clasp your hands together beneath your back, wriggle your shoulders together, and press your arms into the mat. Alternatively, beginners can practise by lowering their legs against a wall.

Take 10-20 slow breaths in the pose, then exhale to release, bending your knees and rolling down slowly, one vertebra at a time.

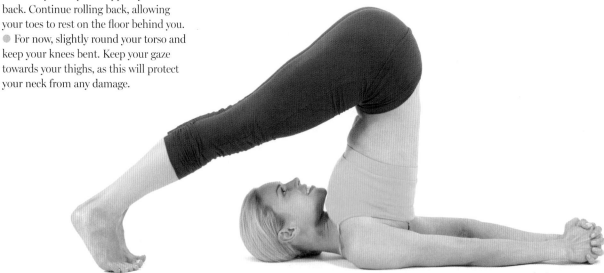

Sivananda benefit

After Shoulderstand, Plough further works your neck and upper back muscles.

Good for:

- *Soothing your nerves*
- *Reducing hypertension*
- *Relieving palpitations*

BRIDGE

Setu bandha sarvangasana

Lie on your back with your legs straight and your arms outstretched, about a foot away from your sides, palms facing upwards. Place the soles of your feet on the floor, directly beneath your knees, hip-distance apart and parallel. Check that your knees are also hip-distance apart.

Take a breath in then, on an exhale, tilt your tailbone upwards as you lift your buttocks off the floor, peeling your spine away from your mat vertebra by vertebra. Interlace your fingers and rest your hands on the floor beneath your torso, arms extended. Snuggle your shoulders together and breathe into your chest.

Roll your shoulders up, back and down, then lengthen the back of your neck. Press your arms into the mat, and focus on grounding through your feet to lift through the heart, making sure your hips remain level.

Take five more deep breaths into your abdomen, then unclasp your fingers and take your arms to your sides. On your next exhale, slowly uncurl your spine, vertebra by vertebra, to release your spine back to the floor. Gently release your legs and place them straight on the floor, feet a comfortable distance apart. Rest for a moment before repeating the pose on the other side

Good for:

- *Relieving fatigue*
- *Toning your back*
- *Opening your chest*

Sivananda benefit

Bridge is a counterpose for Plough that enhances flexibility in your spine.

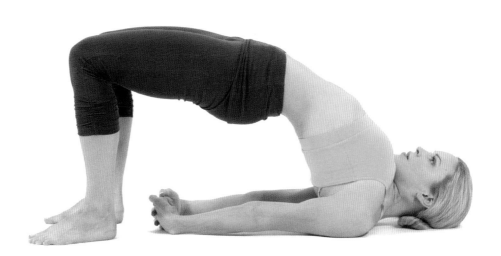

Paschimottanasana

● Sit with your legs straight out in front of you, feet together, ankles flexed and toes pointing to the ceiling. Extend through the balls of your feet, spread your toes and reach through the base of your big and little toes. Lift your arches and draw the outside edges of your feet slightly towards your body. If you have tight hamstrings, sit on a folded blanket, bend your knees or use a strap around the balls of your feet. If your back rounds, sitting on a bolster can be helpful.

● Inhale and take your arms overhead. Exhale as you release your shoulder blades down your back and draw your arms into your shoulder sockets.

● On the next inhalation, root through your sitting bones to extend your spine up out of your pelvis. As you exhale, fold forwards slightly from your hips, keeping your back flat. Pause, then inhale again as you lengthen your spine and, leading from your heart, fold further forwards.

● Continue moving, breath-by-breath, lengthening your front and back spine evenly, as you reach your torso up and forwards to fold over your thighs. As you get lower, release your spine and take your hands either to your shins, outer edges of your feet, or clasp your hands behind your feet.

● Maintain the space around your neck by drawing your shoulders away from your ears, and keep your neck long by extending through your crown and drawing your chin to your chest.

● Breathe deeply and evenly in the pose, feeling the strength of your legs and the expansion in your back body as your spine gently undulates with each in- and out-breath.

● When you feel ready, take a deep inhalation and reach up with your crown as you lead with your heart to return to sitting. Rest for a moment or two with your eyes closed as you allow your body to register the effect of the pose.

Good for:

● *Resting your mind*
● *Relieving stress and anxiety*
● *Reducing fatigue*
● *Easing insomnia*

Sivananda benefit

Opens and stretches the entire back of your body.

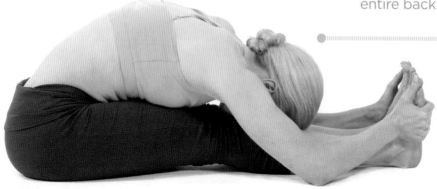

COBRA
Bhujangasana

Lie on your stomach with your forehead resting on the floor. Take a couple of deep breaths, then spread your feet hip-distance apart, ankles straight and toes spread. Straighten your legs, aligning your knees with your middle toes, and engage your inner leg muscles, lifting your inner thighs up and out. Root through your pubic bone.

Place your hands beneath your shoulders, palms facing down, fingers spread and wrist crease parallel with the front edge of your mat. Root through the base of your thumbs and index fingers.

Draw your elbows together and rotate your shoulders up, back and down to create space at the base of your neck, then release your shoulder blades down your back and in towards your spine.

Engage your abdomen and root through your pelvic bone to extend your sacrum to your tailbone. Inhale, and raise your head and shoulders as far as is comfortable by drawing the back of your neck upwards, so your eyes remain looking down. Exhale.

Good for:

- *Strengthening your spine and toning your spinal nerves*
- *Easing tension in your back, shoulders and neck*
- *Helping to relieve stress and fatigue*
- *Opening your heart and lungs*

On an inhale, ground through your hands, as if you were pulling the floor towards you, and feel your chest open as you curl your spine further forwards and up.

Lengthen your spine evenly without compressing the back of your neck or your lumbar spine, and see if you can feel a sense of lightness as you lift your back body.

Breathe normally in the pose for three to five breaths. Slowly and with control, exhale as you lower your body to the floor one vertebra at a time, and rest your head on one side.

Sivananda benefit

Opens your chest area and stimulates your heart.

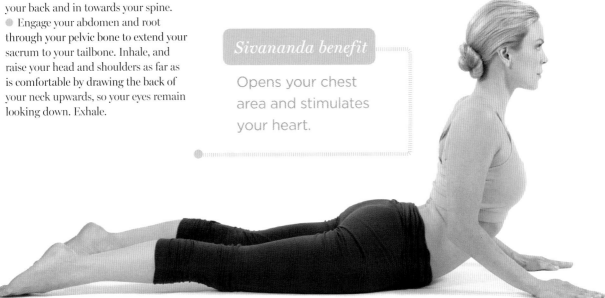

LOCUST
Salabhasana

Lie on your tummy, with your chin resting on your mat, your arms at your sides, palms facing upwards. Turn your big toes towards each other to rotate your thighs inwards and take a few breaths to centre yourself.

On an inhale, draw your navel to your spine and root your pubic bone into the mat as you lift your legs, extending through to your pointed toes. At the same time, raise your head, chest and arms so you're resting on your lower ribs, stomach and lower abdomen. Extend through your arms to your fingertips, imagining you're lifting them up against a weight and bring your shoulder blades in towards your back.

Engage your glutes and reach strongly through your legs, keeping your big toes turning inwards. Lengthen the back of your neck and gaze gently forwards.

Remain in the pose for 30 seconds to one minute, breathing slowly and evenly, then release on an exhale.

Rest your head on your folded arms, face pointing to the side. Then repeat two to three times more.

Good for:

- *Energising*
- *Opening your chest and shoulders*
- *Strengthening your lower back, buttocks, legs and abdomen*

Sivananda benefit

Prepares your body for deeper backbends.

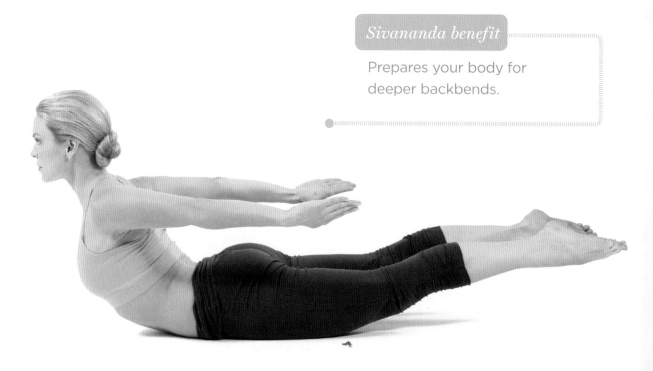

BOW
Dhanurasana

Lie on your stomach with your forehead resting on the floor, arms by your sides, legs straight, feet resting on the tops of your toes. When you feel ready, rotate your shoulders down your spine, then bend your knees and reach back to grasp the outside of each ankle with your hands.

On an inhale, draw your navel in and root your pubic bone into your mat as you lift your chest off it. As you exhale, keeping your arms straight, raise your feet upwards and into your hands.

Externally rotate your upper arms to open your chest further, and keep drawing your shoulders down your back to create space around your ears. Maintain an even curve throughout the length of your spine. Take a couple of breaths here then, on an inhale, lift your chest a little higher, pausing on

Good for:

- *Strengthening your back and legs*
- *Toning your abdominals*
- *Boosting your immunity*
- *Being mentally stimulating*

the exhale. Repeat once or twice more.

Breathe deeply and evenly in the pose, for 10 seconds, gazing softly forwards. If comfortable, gradually build up to 30 seconds, while working on bringing your knees, feet and ankles closer together.

To come down, on an exhale, gently release your feet, stretch your legs and lower your arms and legs to the floor then rest your head on one side.

If you only stayed up for a few seconds, you can repeat the pose a few times, then lie on your stomach, resting your head on your folded arms.

Sivananda benefit

Works your entire back simultaneously.

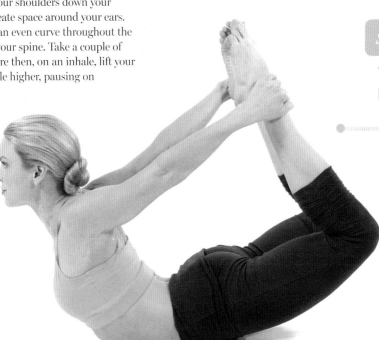

Marichyasana C

Sit with your legs out in front of you, feet together, ankles flexed and toes pointing to the ceiling. Rest your hands or fingertips on the floor beside your hips, fingers spread, fingertips facing forwards. Close your eyes to become centred.

When ready, extend through the balls of your feet, spread your toes and reach through the base of your big and little toes. Lift your arches and draw the outside edges of your feet to your body. Breathe.

Bend your left knee and place your foot a hand's distance from your left thigh, knee directly above your ankle. Root though your big and little toes and the centre of your heel, and lift the inner arch.

Raise your right arm overhead, then as you exhale, lower your arm and place your outer right elbow against your outer left knee, forearm vertical and fingers pointing to the ceiling. Inhale, and as you exhale, twist your body towards the left.

Breathe softly and deeply, filling your abdomen and ribcage, for up to one minute. As you root down through your sitting bones, feel the corresponding lift through your torso. Lengthen your spine on each inhalation, twist a little more on each exhalation, using the resistance of your forearm against your knee to help.

Keep your core active, by drawing your navel to your spine, opening your chest and drawing your shoulders down your back. If comfortable, turn your head to gaze over your left shoulder. Breathe, and be aware of the sensations you're experiencing.

When you're ready, inhale, then exhale to return to centre and pause before twisting to the right as a brief counter pose, then repeat on the other side.

Good for:

- *Lengthening your spine*
- *Deeply releasing your back, shoulders and neck*
- *Aiding detoxification*
- *Nourishing your spinal nerves*

Sivananda benefit

After bending forwards and backwards, this pose works on maintaining sideways flexibility in your spine.

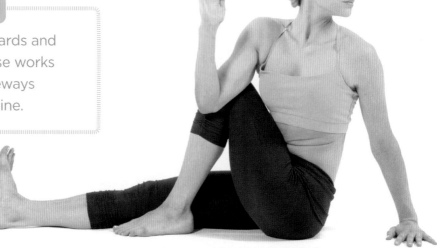

GARLAND
Malasana

Centre yourself in Mountain pose (p36), then, when you feel ready, step your feet wider than hip-width apart. Inhale, and on an exhale, gently crouch down into a low squat, taking your hands to the floor in front of you.

Turn your feet out, so your knees are over your toes, then lower your heels, taking your feet as far apart as is needed so that your heels can anchor firmly into the ground. If your heels still don't touch the floor place a folded blanket beneath them to support you.

Lift your hands into prayer position and let your tailbone release to your mat.

Press your palms together as you root through your feet, and push your upper arms into your inner thighs and your thighs into your arms. This will help you lift out of your pelvis to lengthen through your spine.

Draw your shoulder blades down your back and let your chest expand. Take five to 10 deep breaths into your belly.

When you're ready to come out, release your hands and come to a comfortable seated position for a few breaths while you register the effects of the pose.

Good for:

- *Relieving tension in your back*
- *Loosening your hips*
- *Calming yourself*
- *Aiding your focus*

Sivananda benefit

Aids mental balance and tranquility as a preparation for Crow pose.

Uttanasana

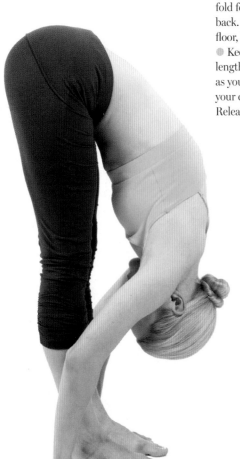

- From Mountain pose (p36), with your feet hip-distance apart, take your hands to your hips and, on an inhale, root through your feet to lengthen your torso away from your pelvis.
- Exhale, bend your knees slightly and fold forwards from your hips with a flat back. When your spine is parallel to the floor, let your pelvis come into neutral.
- Keeping your knees bent, inhale to lengthen your spine once more, then, as you exhale, continue folding and allow your chest to rest on your thighs. Release your arms and rest your

hands on your shins, ankles or the floor.
- If it feels comfortable, straighten your legs, keeping a microbend in your knees, then allow your upper body to relax fully. Take your tailbone towards the ceiling, and your head closer to the floor.
- On each in-breath, feel your spine lengthening; on each out-breath, fold a little deeper. If you wish to deepen the stretch, rest the backs of your hands on the floor and slide them under your feet, fingertips leading. Press the soles of your feet onto the palms of your hands.
- Consciously surrender, breathing softly and evenly for several breaths, then inhale to gently uncurl your spine to return to standing.

Good for:

- *Calming your nervous system*
- *Relieving fatigue*
- *Stretching your entire back body*
- *Regulating blood pressure*

VARIATION

Half-standing forward fold

From Standing forward fold, knees bent or straight, place your hands a few inches in front of your feet. Inhale as you lengthen your crown away from your tailbone to come up to a flat back. Root through your hands and feet and draw your shoulder blades down your spine. Take five deep breaths and release back into Standing forward fold.

Sivananda benefit

Strengthens your spine and legs and increases flexibility in both.

TRIANGLE
Utthita trikonasana

Stand sideways on the centre of your mat and take a moment to arrive in your body, breathing deeply into your belly. When ready, step your feet a leg's-length apart.

Turn your left foot out 90 degrees and your right foot in 15 degrees. Align your heels (or left heel to right instep), then root down through your big and little toes, the centre of your heels and the outer edge of your right foot. Breathe.

Place your hands on your hips and tilt your left hip down and right hip back and up. On an inhale, extend your arms out to shoulder height. As you exhale, keep your arms parallel to the floor as you reach your left hand outwards as far as is comfortable, before releasing it down to rest where it lands, on your calf or ankle.

On your next inhale, float your right arm overhead and rotate to open your chest, so your right shoulder is above the left and your arms are in a straight line. Let your gaze rest on the floor, directly ahead or, if comfortable for your neck, turn your head to look up at your top hand.

Breathe into the pose, making micro-adjustments, until you feel rooted but

open, using your in-breath to ground through your feet and lengthen your side body, and your out-breath to release further into the twist. Rest in your final position for 30 seconds to two minutes, breathing deeply into your belly.

When ready, root through your feet and inhale up to standing, then exhale as you lower your arms and step your feet together. Pause to register the effects of the pose, then repeat on the other side.

Good for:

- *Relieving stiffness in your legs, hips and neck*
- *Relieving tension in your back*
- *Opening your side body/ improving your breathing*
- *Easing menstrual symptoms*

Sivananda benefit

Increases flexibility in your legs, hips and shoulders.

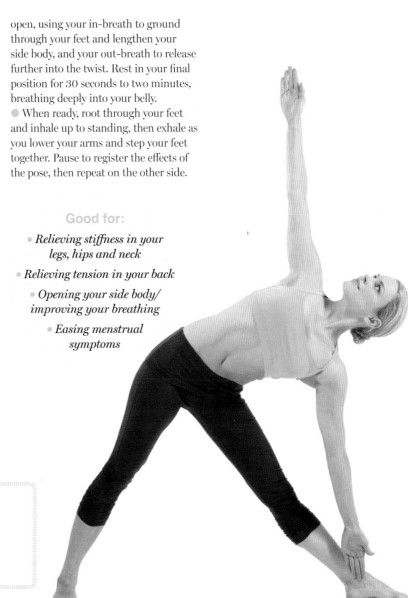

THE SIVANANDA
sequence

Boost your wellbeing

This sequence is based around the poses in a traditional Sivananda class – with one or two modifications to enable everyone to enjoy the benefits – and will give you a good feel for the style. If you've been practising yoga for less than a year, do four to six slow Sun salutes (p24), depending on your energy. Those with more experience can do eight to 10 rounds. Remember to include Savasana or Relaxation pose (p47) after every pose, as it is integral to creating the sense of inner peace that Sivananda is renowned for.

1 Headstand (p72)
Followed by Relaxation pose

2 Shoulder stand (p73)
Followed by Relaxation pose

3 Plough (p74)
Followed by Relaxation pose

4 Bridge (p75)
Followed by Relaxation pose

5 Seated forward fold (p76)
Followed by Relaxation pose

6 Cobra (p77)
Followed by Relaxation pose

7 Locust (p78)
Followed by Relaxation pose

8 Bow (p79)
Followed by Relaxation pose

9 Seated twist (p80)
Followed by Relaxation pose

10 Garland (p81)
Followed by Relaxation pose

11 Standing forward fold (p82)
Followed by Relaxation pose

12 Triangle (p83)
Followed by 10 to 15 minutes in Relaxation pose

The moves

START

Savasana
5 minutes
Single leg lifts and Double leg lifts (p70)
Kapalabhati *(p71)*

Sun salute I *(p24)*

① ② ③ ④

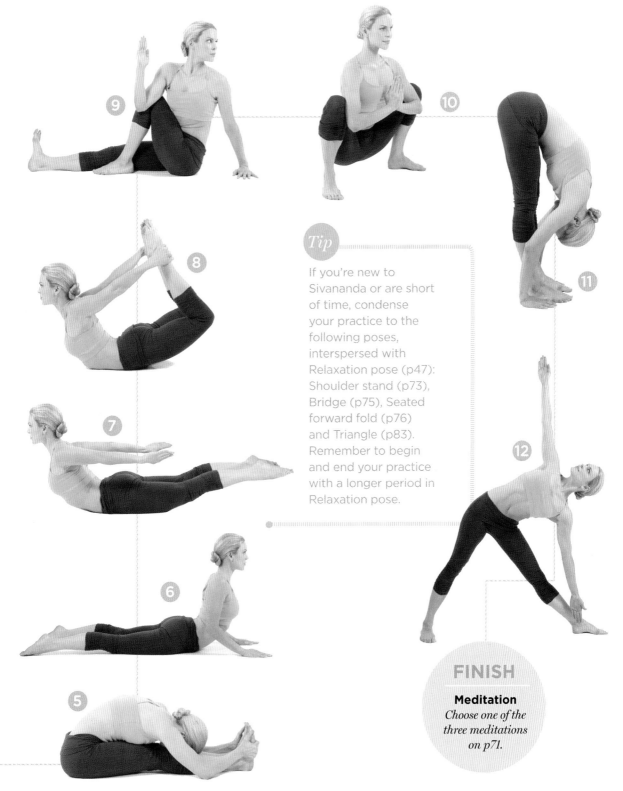

Tip

If you're new to
Sivananda or are short
of time, condense
your practice to the
following poses,
interspersed with
Relaxation pose (p47):
Shoulder stand (p73),
Bridge (p75), Seated
forward fold (p76)
and Triangle (p83).
Remember to begin
and end your practice
with a longer period in
Relaxation pose.

FINISH

Meditation
*Choose one of the
three meditations
on p71.*

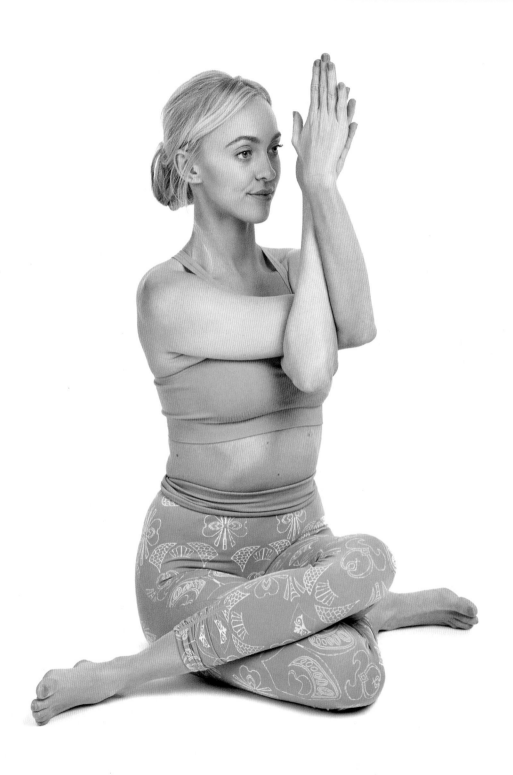

Yin

Now you've worked on your **alignment**, *learnt some challenging poses and experienced how to put postures together in a flow, it's time to slow things down. In Yin yoga, you'll mostly be* **lying or sitting** *on your mat, holding poses for longer periods of time – up to five minutes or sometimes even more. It's an ideal style of yoga to practise when you're feeling tired, if your mind is racing or you're feeling overstimulated. Not only will it help* **relax** *your system and calm your nerves, you'll find it gently* **energising** *too. You can also practise Yin when you want to increase your flexibility as it's a style that specifically* **targets** *your joints and deeper connective tissues in your lower body. Just remember to balance* **calming** *Yin sessions with a more active yang sequence such as Iyengar or Vinyasa a couple of times a week.*

INTRODUCTION TO
Yin

A relatively new form of yoga, Yin owes its existence largely to Paulie Zink, whose version of Taoist yoga became popular in the 1970s and has since been developed by teachers Bernie Clark, Paul Grilley and Sarah Powers to become the form we know today. Based on the Chinese concepts of yin and yang - yin being cool, solid, stable and internal, yang being hot, active, moving and external - it focuses on stretching the yin tissues of the body, such as tendons, ligaments and fascia. While yang tissues –muscles – give your body strength, it's the yin tissues that give it flexibility.

Yin postures also affect the meridians, or energy channels, in your body. When a meridian is blocked, energy or chi, cannot flow freely in your body, and can lead to ill health. If you have any of the following issues, practising poses associated with the relevant meridian may be helpful.

- **Liver meridian**: low back or abdominal pain, mental health issues
- **Gall bladder meridian**: headache, blurred vision, pain along the side of your body
- **Kidney meridian**: kidney issues, gynae problems, lung or throat symptoms
- **Urinary bladder meridian**: head or back pain, mental health issues
- **Spleen meridian**: digestive issues, unnecessary anxiety
- **Stomach meridian**: bloating, vomiting, pain in the nose, mouth, teeth

BEFORE YOU BEGIN

It's a good idea to spend a few moments setting an intention for your practice. A few quiet breaths with closed eyes will help you tune in to your deepest need and help you stay committed to supporting this aspect of yourself while you work with the asanas. Aim to take slow, even breaths throughout your practice. Some people like to use Ocean breath, a very gentle form of Ujjayi (p35), and remember to breathe into any tight areas to help soften the tension held there.

As your muscles need to be cooler when doing a Yin practice – if your muscles are warm, the stress will be placed on them and not on your tendons and fascia (the connective tissue surrounding your muscles) – there's no warm-up for these sessions. If you'd like a bit more movement, but still want the benefits and calming energy of a Yin session, you could do one of the Moon salutes (p28 and p30) after your practice or on alternate days.

> " *Yin yoga focuses on stretching the yin tissues of the body, such as tendons, ligaments and fascia* "

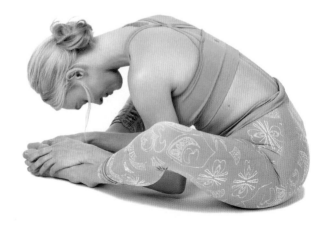

Pranayama

HAMSA MANTRA

■ In yogic philosophy, a mantra is a sound or group of sounds believed to have the power to create change or transformation. Bija mantras, or seed mantras, are said to activate energy centres in the body, known as chakras, to help bring you into a state of balance. In this practice we use the 'ham' seed mantra, associated with the throat chakra.

■ Spend a few moments breathing in to your belly and, when you feel centred, begin. Inhale, then as you exhale slowly, almost silently say the word 'ham'; as you slowly inhale, say the word 'sa'. Close your eyes and breathe in this way for a couple of minutes. As you become more familiar with the technique, notice whether you can sense any difference in your body or energy on the inhale and the exhale.

■ Try reversing the process, chanting 'ham' as you inhale, 'sa' as you exhale. Does this feel different? Does one feel more energising, the other more calming? If you find the technique beneficial, you can use it on or off your mat when you want to change the way you feel.

SPINAL BREATHING

■ Sit comfortably with your eyes closed and take a few deep breaths to centre yourself. When ready, take your attention to your heart area. On your next inhalation, imagine travelling down your spine to your tailbone, noticing any sensations – heat, aching, tightness. There may be places of numbness where you sense nothing at all. As you exhale, mentally trace your spine from your tailbone to your heart. Continue breathing like this for a few rounds, moving and breathing slowly and mindfully. Don't worry if you don't feel anything, it takes time to build your sensitivity. Just notice your experience and, over time, it will grow and develop.

Meditation

OPENING MEDITATION

■ Sit comfortably or lie on your back and spend a few moments to arrive in your body. Take a few deep inhalations, releasing your out breath with a sigh through an open mouth. When you feel more settled and present, bring your attention to the area below your navel and gently notice the rise and fall of your belly as you breathe. There's no need to change anything, just observe the sensations you're experiencing.

■ After a minute or two, start to notice other physical sensations in your body, the feel of the air or your clothes on your skin, the pressure of your body resting on the floor beneath you or sounds entering your awareness. When you feel ready, move your attention to your heart area and begin to become aware of any emotions you're feeling. Are you hesitant, bored or impatient to start moving? Again, don't try to change anything, just be a witness to what is already present within you.

■ Finally, let your awareness rest on the point between the centre of your eyes, the bridge of the nose. Notice any thoughts that are coming in and out of your consciousness. No thought is good or bad, so try not to judge any of them, just notice them arrive, accept their presence and let them drift away. After a couple of minutes, take your attention back to your heart, rest there a moment or two, then gently open your eyes.

SHOELACE

● From all-fours, lift your right knee, take it back slightly and cross it over your left calf to place it outside your left shin. Spread your feet away from each other, then exhale as you gently lower your bottom to sit between your feet.

● Root evenly through both sitting bones. If one side doesn't touch the floor, place a folded blanket or thin block beneath it. Holding a foot in each hand, guide your feet as far forwards as is comfortable, keeping one knee above the other. If your bottom leg is uncomfortable keep your bottom leg extended in front of you.

● Take a couple of breaths to acclimatise to the stretch. Then root through your sitting bones as you open your chest, lengthen the back of your neck and lift through your crown on the in-breath, allowing your weight to sink down on the out-breath.

● Softly inhale as you float your arms out to the sides, shoulder height. Exhale and cross your arms in front of you with your left elbow on top of your right. Then intertwine your forearms to bring your palms together, fingertips pointing up and thumbs facing you. Gently close your eyes.

● Take a few deep abdominal breaths, expanding into your back and side body, then let your breath find its natural rhythm. Settle into a sense of stillness, resting in the pose for up to three to five minutes.

● Gently release your arms and, with great care, your legs, then pause for a moment in a comfortable seated position, before repeating on the other side.

Good for:

- *Removing tension from your shoulders*
- *Opening your hips*
- *Calming anxiety*
- *Opening your lower back (see tip)*

Meridians

Liver and gall bladder

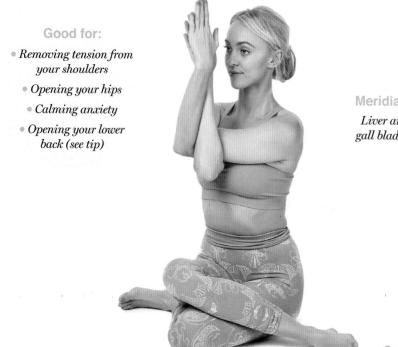

Tip

To release your back muscles, fold forwards, extending your arms straight in front of you and resting your palms on the floor.

SLEEPING SWAN

Come onto all-fours, with your hands shoulder-distance apart, about a handspan in front of your shoulders. Bring your right knee forwards and place it behind and outside your right wrist. Initially, your right shin bone is at about a 45-degree angle, with your right heel beneath your left hip. As you progress, place your shin parallel to the front edge of your mat for a stronger hip opener.

Slide your left leg straight behind you and rest on the centre of your front thigh. Draw your right hip back and your left hip forwards to square your pelvis. If the thigh of your bent leg doesn't reach the floor, place a block or folded blanket beneath your hip, so your hips are fully supported.

Inhale and root through your hands to lengthen your spine, extending through your crown then, on an exhale, fold forwards over your bent leg. Place your forehead on the back of your hands or rest it on a bolster.

This is a strong hip opener – direct your breath towards tension in your hip to help disperse the intensity. Breathe softly and deeply for one to three minutes.

When you're ready to come out, inhale and root through your hands to come up and gently release your legs. Repeat on the other side, then rest in child's pose.

Good for:

- *Externally rotating your front hip*
- *Opening your back hip flexor*
- *Stretching your back quads*

Meridians

Gall bladder and liver

Tip

Check that the foot of your back leg is directly behind your hip, and the front of your hip is facing your mat.

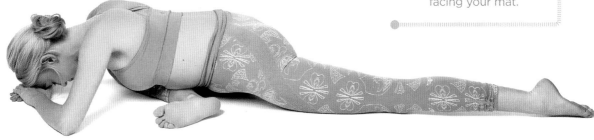

HAPPY BABY

● Lie on your back and take a moment to centre yourself. Take three deep breaths, releasing any tension on the exhale.

● When you feel ready, bend your knees deeply, take hold of your outer feet with each hand and open your knees, allowing them to release down towards your armpits.

● Flex your ankles, with the soles facing the ceiling, and bring your calves to vertical. Feel the stretch

and deep release in your lower back.

● Tuck in your chin to lengthen your neck, and draw your shoulders down your spine to create space around your neck. Reach your tailbone forwards to lengthen your spine.

● If you're pulling with your arms, stay in the pose for two minutes. If your arms are relaxed, you can rest for up to five minutes, breathing slowly and deeply, then rock gently from side to side before releasing your feet to the floor.

Good for:

● *Relieving stress*

● *Opening your inner and outer thighs*

● *Releasing & decompressing your sacroiliac joint*

● *Uplifting*

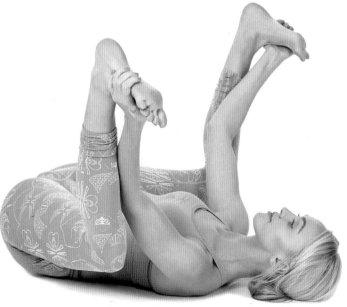

Meridians

Liver, kidney and bladder

Tip

If your hips are tight, wrap a strap around the balls of your feet, holding one end in each hand, and gradually walk your hands up the strap as your flexibility increases.

DRAGON FLYING LOW

● From Crescent pose (p56), heel/toe your right foot towards the edge of your mat, then place your hands to the inside of your front foot.

● Check that your right knee is directly above your ankle, hug it into the mid-line and ground through the base of your big and little toes.

● Extend through your back heel and keep your thigh lifted then, one arm at a time, lower onto your forearms, fingers spread and middle finger pointed towards the front of your mat. Check your elbows are directly beneath your shoulders.

● Ground through your forearms so you don't sink into your shoulders and draw

your shoulderblades down your back to create space around you ears. Lightly engage your abdomen, breathing deeply into your belly or directing your breath into any areas of tightness in your groin, and rest in the pose for three to five minutes. Release on an exhale and repeat on the other side.

Good for:

- *Opening your hips deeply*
- *Stretching your quads and hip flexors*
- *Opening your groin*
- *Easing sciatica*

Tip

Ease into the pose by resting your forearms on a bolster or block, removing them as your flexibility increases.

Meridians

Kidney, stomach, spleen, liver and gall bladder

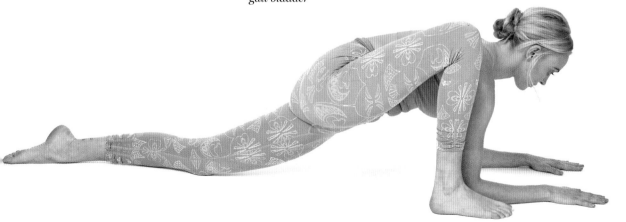

SADDLE

● Kneel up on your mat with your knees slightly apart, tops of your feet flat on the floor, and gently ease your buttocks down between your feet. If you have tight ankles, place a cushion beneath them, and if your knees are uncomfortable, place a rolled blanket behind them.

● Take your hands behind you and rest your fingertips on the floor, leaning backwards as you do so. Arch your upper back, and tilt your tailbone back towards your lower spine, to deeply arch your back.

● If not too much of a strain on your quadriceps (front thighs), gently lower onto your forearms. Allow your knees to remain apart, to avoid stressing the joints, and rest in the pose for one to five minutes. If comfortable, you can lie back on your mat or on a bolster and take your arms overhead to stretch out your shoulders.

● To come out of the posture, gently engage your abdominals, and come back to keeling. Rest for a moment or two lying in Relaxation pose (p47) and clench and release your kneecaps to relieve any tension. Draw your knees to your chest, then roll over onto your side to come up to sitting.

Meridians

Stomach, spleen, bladder and kidneys

Good for:

● *Opening your hip flexors*
● *Stretching your quads*
● *Rotating your hips internally*

Tip

For sensitive knees, keep one leg straight and the other bent, switching sides after a few minutes. Over time you'll be able to practise with both knees bent.

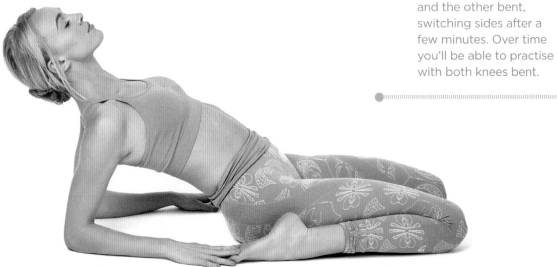

CAT PULLING ITS TAIL

● Lie on your back, knees bent and feet flat on the floor close to your buttocks. Raise your hips off the ground and shift your buttocks a few inches to your right as you lower your hips back to your mat.
● Straighten your left leg only and, pressing into the ground through your right foot, raise your hips once more and shift your buttocks further to the right. Twist at the waist to roll onto your left hip, so your right hip is stacked directly over your left hip, all the time keeping your back and shoulders flat on the mat.

● Bring your left arm into cactus arms (pictured) and straighten your right leg. Bend your left knee so your foot reaches towards your buttocks and grasp hold of your toes with your right hand. Pull your hand towards you at the same time as you pull your foot away from your hand. This will create a deep stretch in your left quadriceps.
● Rest here for three to five minutes, then release your left foot and roll onto your stomach. Pause for a moment before repeating on the other side.

Good for:

● *Relaxing deeply*
● *Aiding insomnia*
● *Stretching your quads*
● *Easing tension in your lower back*

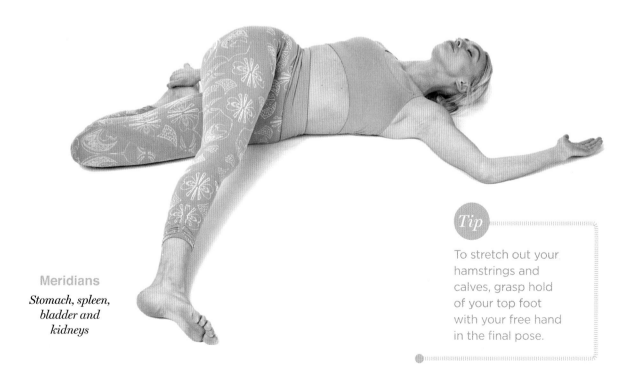

Meridians

Stomach, spleen, bladder and kidneys

Tip

To stretch out your hamstrings and calves, grasp hold of your top foot with your free hand in the final pose.

BUTTERFLY

Sit on your mat, checking that your weight is evenly distributed between your sitting bones. Bend your knees and bring the soles of your feet together, then let them fall out to the side like a butterfly's wings.

After a moment or two, slide your feet forwards to make a diamond shape with your legs.

Grasp your feet with your hands and fold forwards, letting your weight come onto the front of your sitting bones as you allow your spine to gently drape forwards. Let your neck release and your forehead drop towards your hands.

Rest for a while here then, as you feel your muscles soften and release, sink a little deeper into the pose. If your groin feels tight, rest your knees on a block.

Spend three to five minutes, or longer if comfortable, breathing slowly and deeply into your belly, then inhale and engage your abdomen to come back up to sitting.

Slowly stretch your legs in front of you and lean back on your hands, gently arching your back as a counterpose to the forward bend.

Good for:

- *Regulating your periods*
- *Releasing tension in your spine*
- *Loosening your lower back*
- *Calming your brain*

Meridians

Gall bladder and urinary bladder

Tip

If your back feels strained, sit on a block or bolster.

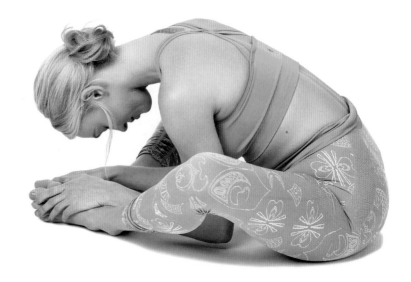

SNAIL

Lie on your back with your knees bent, feet flat on the floor and your arms by your sides, palms down. Take a few breaths into your belly to quieten your mind.

Bring your knees to your chest, then straighten your legs to take your feet up towards the ceiling.

Take a deep breath then, on an exhale, root through your hands to lift your legs up and over your head to the floor behind you, knees slightly bent, toes tucked under. At the same time, take your hands to your side ribs to support your back.

Stay here for a few breaths, with your back slightly curved. Unlike the traditional yang pose, Plough (p74), this yin version has a soft rounded spine. Straighten your legs and reach through your heels.

If comfortable here, release your hands and extend your arms, palms facing upwards and breathe slowly and evenly into your belly for three to five minutes.

To come out of the pose, raise your feet and uncurl your spine, releasing it one vertebra at a time to the floor until you're flat on your back. Pause for a moment or two, then come into Bridge (p75), to realign your spine.

Good for:

- *Deeply releasing your spine*
- *Alleviating fatigue*
- *Calming your brain*
- *Easing insomnia*

Tip

If your feet can't reach the floor behind you, rest them on a bolster or the seat of a chair. Alternatively, do Happy baby (p92) instead.

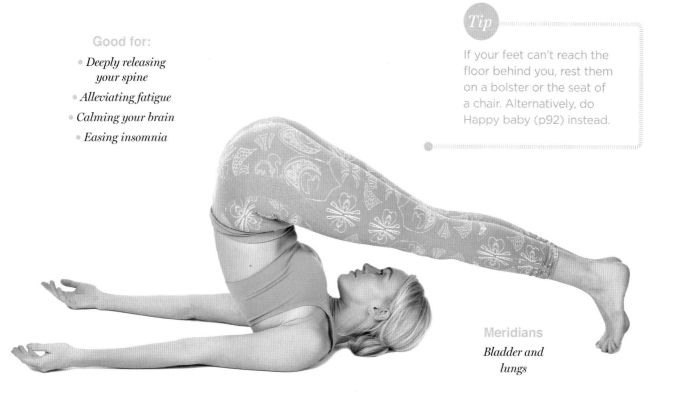

Meridians
Bladder and lungs

SPHINX

Lie on your stomach with your feet shoulder-width apart, resting on the tops of your toes. Relax your buttocks and legs.

Take your upper body weight onto your forearms, keeping them parallel and your elbows shoulder-width apart. Spread your fingertips and root through the base of your fingers and thumbs.

Press your weight into your forearms so you don't sink into your shoulders, and draw your shoulder blades down your back. Gently engage your inner thighs, but allow your belly to sink towards the floor. Keep your neck in line with your spine and gaze softly forwards, or, if comfortable, let it reach back slightly and look upwards.

Rest in the pose for three to five minutes, then lower back to the mat on an exhale.

Good for:

- *Toning your spine*
- *Stimulating your lower back*
- *Stimulating your thyroid (when your neck is released back)*

Tip

Rest your forearms on a bolster to raise your chest higher and to deepen the backbend.

Meridians

Bladder, kidneys, stomach and spleen

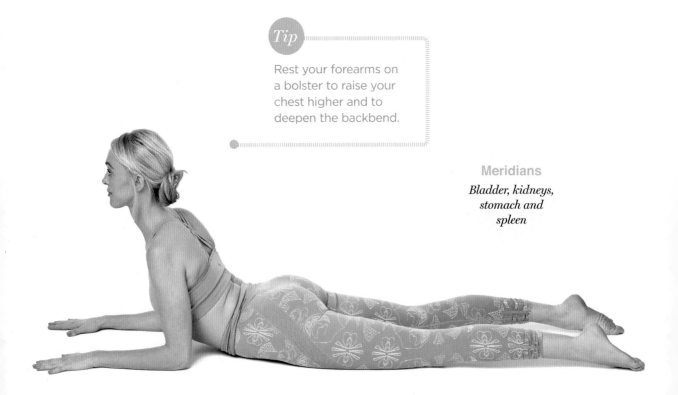

TWISTED DRAGON

● From Crescent (p56), heel/toe your right foot towards the edge of your mat, then place your hands to the inside of your front foot.

● Check that your right knee is directly above your ankle, hug it into the mid-line and ground through the base of your big and little toes.

● Inhale, and gently engage your abdomen as you lift your torso and bring your hands to prayer position. On an exhale, twist to the right, hooking your left elbow outside your right thigh. Extend your heart forwards and to the right while simultaneously drawing your shoulders down your back. Lightly draw your navel to your spine.

● Rest in the pose for three to five minutes before releasing on an exhale. Repeat on the other side.

Good for:

- *As for Dragon flying low (p93), plus:*
- *Aiding your digestion*
- *Opening your chest*
- *Stretching your upper back muscles*

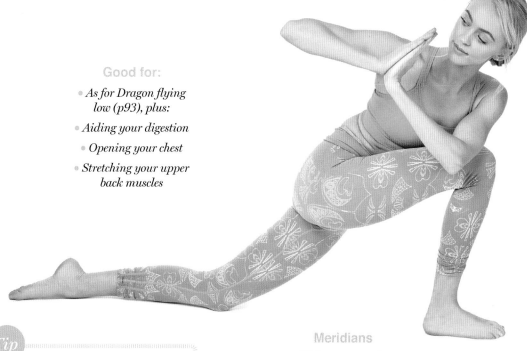

Tip

If you have sensitive knees, place a folded blanket beneath your back knee or rest your shin on a bolster.

Meridians

Kidneys, stomach, spleen, liver and gall bladder

MOUNTAIN BROOK

WHAT YOU NEED: BOLSTER, BLANKETS, EYE BAG (OPTIONAL)

● Fold two blankets into strips and another into a rectangle, rolling up one edge to make a support for your neck. Arrange the props on your mat as in the image, then lie on your back, with the blankets and bolster supporting you.

● Make any adjustments you need, decreasing or increasing the height of the blankets, to ensure your neck is fully supported, your head tilting gently back and your chest open, but not strained.

● Extend your arms to the sides, palms facing upwards and gently close your eyes, using an eye bag if you wish.

● Spend a few moments breathing into your chest area, allowing your ribs to expand and your shoulders to release into the floor. On each exhale, let your body feel heavier and heavier as it sinks into the mat.

● Allow your breath to return to normal, then remain in the pose for up to five minutes. When you feel ready, remove your eye bag, softly stretch your whole body and gently roll onto your side before coming up to sitting.

Good for:

• *Opening your shoulders and chest*

• *Aiding breathing*

• *Reducing fatigue*

• *Lifting your mood*

Tip

For a deeper chest lift and shoulder opener, replace the blankets beneath your back with a round bolster.

Meridian

Heart

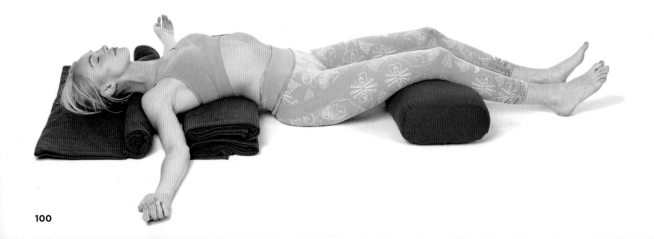

RELAXATION WITH BOLSTER

WHAT YOU NEED: BOLSTER, BLANKETS, EYE BAG (OPTIONAL)

◉ Place a bolster crosswise about a quarter of the way down your mat, and roll one side of a folded blanket at the other end. Have another blanket and an eye bag close by.

◉ Rather than lean back to lie down, which places a strain on your abdomen, from kneeling, lower down onto your right buttock and place your right hand out to the side. Use your hands and forearms to help you lower down onto your right side, then roll over onto your back.

◉ Take your arms to your sides, palms facing up, and bring your chin lower than your forehead to quieten the frontal lobes of your brain. Cover your eyes with an eye bag and your body with a blanket.

◉ Breathing softly and deeply into your belly, scan your body from head to toe, consciously letting go of any tension on an out-breath. Relax your temples

and release your lower jaw. Lengthen the back of your neck and let go of any tension around your lips. Let your eyeballs sink into your eye sockets, and your eyelids be heavy.

◉ Continue travelling down your body, letting your muscles melt into your bones and your bones sink into the mat. Let your thoughts recede and your mind become still, resting here for up to 20 minutes.

◉ When ready to come out of the pose, take your attention to your breath, then bring some movement back to your body. Wriggle your fingers and toes, take your arms overhead and stretch from your hands to your feet. Bring the soles of your feet onto the bolster, take your hips to the left and roll to your right. Rest in a foetal position for a few breaths, then press your left hand into the floor to help you come up to a sitting position.

Good for:
- *Releasing muscular tension*
- *Reducing fatigue*
- *Improving sleep*
- *Lowering blood pressure and your heart rate*

Tip

If your mind starts to wander, bring your attention back to your breath. If it helps, count your breath, saying inwardly 'in one, out one', 'in two, out two', and so on. After a while, you can just say 'one' on the out breath, 'two' on the next out breath.

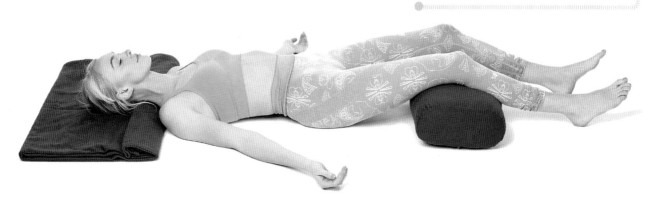

YIN SEQUENCE FOR
hips and legs

Improve your **flexibility**

You don't need to warm your body in Yin yoga as your muscles need to be cool in order for the stress of working in the pose to be placed on your connective tissues and not your muscles for maximum flexibility benefits . However, before you begin your session, quietening your mind, tuning in to how you're feeling physically and emotionally, and understanding what you'd like to receive from your practice will enhance its benefits. If you feel any tightness in your joints, direct your breath towards the area using a very gentle form of Ujjayi breathing, known in Yin circles as Ocean breath. Unless otherwise stated, rest in each pose for up to five minutes.

1 Shoelace (p90)
Three to five minutes each side

1 Sleeping swan (p91)
One to three minutes each side

3 Happy baby (p92)

4 Dragon flying low (p93)

5 Saddle (p94)
Up to two minutes

6 Cat pulling its tail (p95)
Up to four minutes each side

7 Relaxation with bolster (p101)
Up to 20 minutes

The moves

START
Warm-up
Set your intention (p89)

Meditation
Opening meditation (p89)

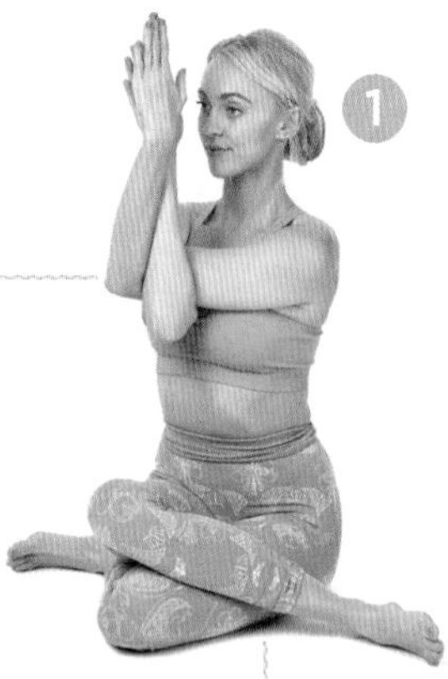

1

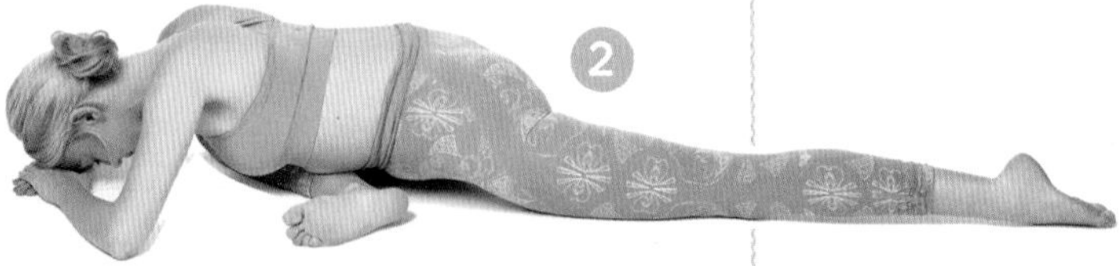

2

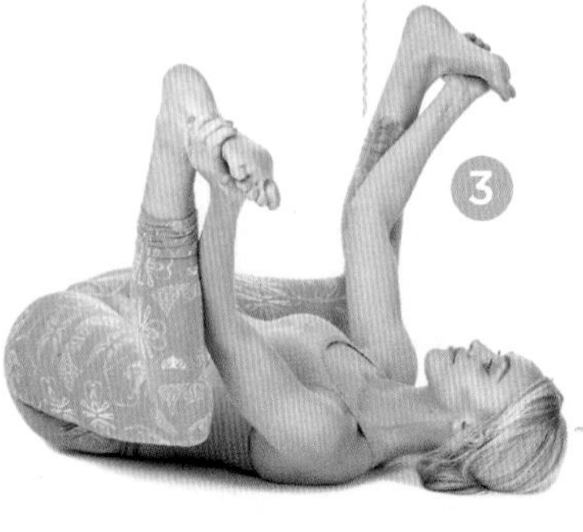

3

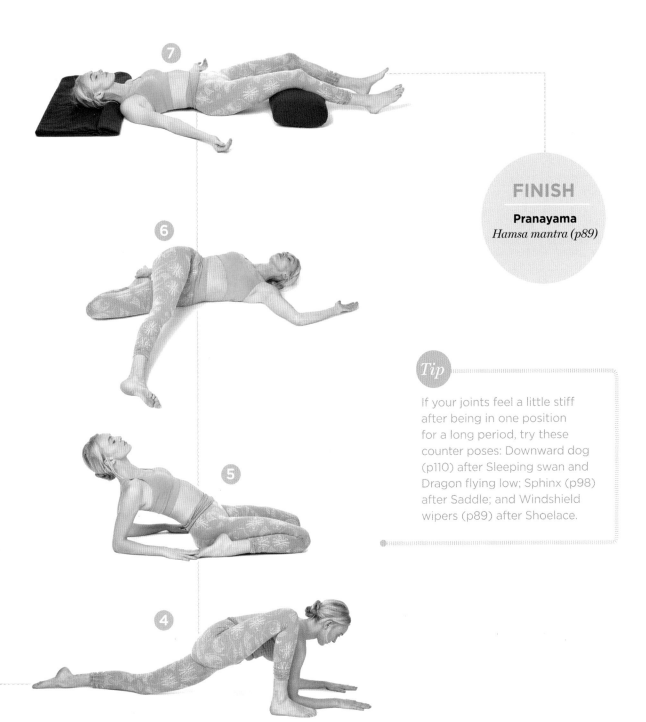

FINISH

Pranayama
Hamsa mantra (p89)

Tip

If your joints feel a little stiff after being in one position for a long period, try these counter poses: Downward dog (p110) after Sleeping swan and Dragon flying low; Sphinx (p98) after Saddle; and Windshield wipers (p89) after Shoelace.

YIN SEQUENCE FOR
spine and shoulders

Ease muscle **tension**

Working with your spine is central to Yin yoga. Not only will it improve your flexibility and spinal-disc health, it also helps to clear stagnation, crucial for allowing a free flow of energy through your central nadi, the shushumna. This sequence also includes poses to release muscular tension in the area between your shoulder blades and to open your chest to counteract hours spent hunched over a computer. Unless otherwise stated, rest in the pose for three to five minutes, using a gentle ocean breath.

1 Butterfly (p96)

2 Shoelace (p90)
Three to five minutes each side

3 Snail (p97)

4 Sphinx (p98)

5 Twisted dragon (p99)
Three to five minutes each side

6 Mountain brook (p100)

7 Relaxation with bolster (p101)
Up to 20 minutes

The moves

START

Warm-up
Set your intention (p89)

Meditation
Opening meditation (p89)

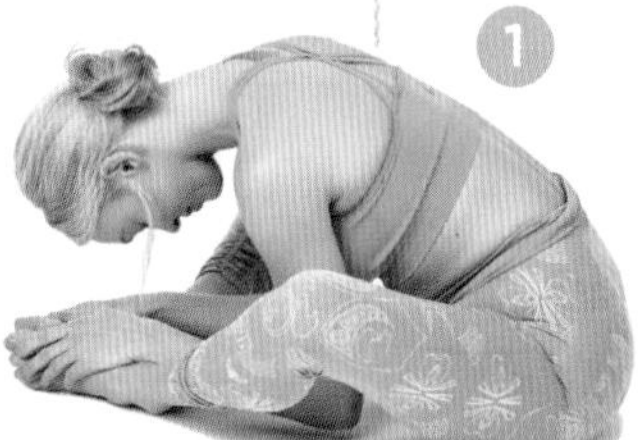

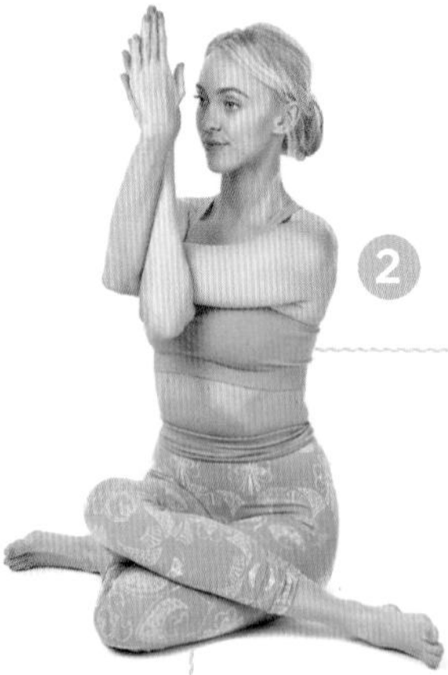

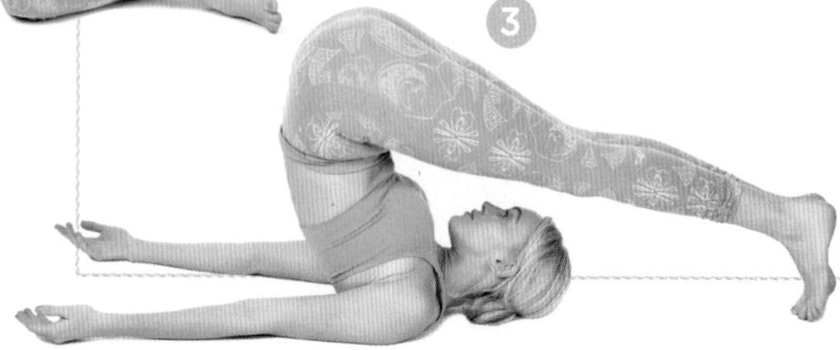

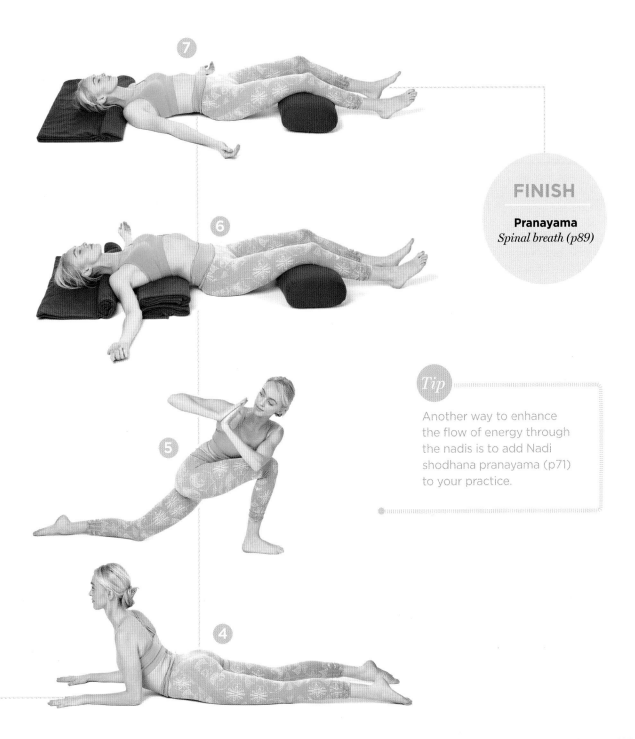

FINISH

Pranayama
Spinal breath (p89)

Tip

Another way to enhance the flow of energy through the nadis is to add Nadi shodhana pranayama (p71) to your practice.

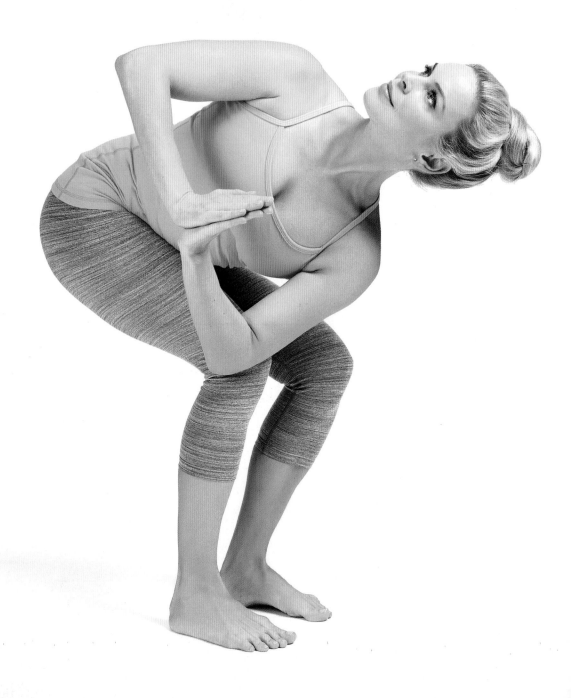

Restorative

Well done on reaching the last chapter of this book! You'll now be familiar with a variety of yoga styles and have built a large store of postures to draw on. Here, we introduce yet another style of yoga, one that will enable you to deeply rest and **nourish your system** in times of stress, whether physical or mental. You'll already know many of the postures from earlier in the book, but here we've given them a restorative twist, to **minimise stress** on your system and enable you to let go completely, so your nervous system can **replenish** itself and begin to heal. You'll be using lots of props to support your body as fully as possible, and resting in poses for up to 20 minutes. All you need to do is surrender to the pose and bathe in the feelings of **release** and **calm** that it brings. Enjoy!

INTRODUCTION TO
Restorative

Restorative yoga owes a big debt to BKS Iyengar, and his influence is especially seen in the use of props, long-held poses and the therapeutic use of postures, but it was a student of his, Judith Lasater, who is most strongly associated with the current popularity of the style. Her book *Relax and Renew* (Rodmell Press, £19.99) was the first solely devoted to the supported yoga poses and breathing techniques of Restorative yoga.

The aim of the style is to help counteract the side effects of everyday stresses, bringing relief from issues such as headache, migraine, anxiety, palpitations and insomnia; in fact, anything that indicates a stressed-out nervous system. Restorative yoga activates your parasympathetic nervous system: the rest and digest system that helps slow the breath and heart rate, and replenish vital organs with a fresh supply of blood, oxygen and nutrients. You can help it do its job better by working mindfully with your breath in your Restorative practice. Notice if you're breathing deeply into your belly or simply taking shallow chest breaths (often the first sign of a stress response), and aim to maintain a steady, even, full abdominal breath. Some people can find the long-held postures and silence that ensues a little uncomfortable. If you experience this, simply bring your attention back to your breath and you'll feel more grounded.

> *It aims to bring relief from anything that indicates a stressed-out nervous system*

BEFORE YOU BEGIN

- Some people like to play music while they're doing Restorative yoga, others prefer silence. Experiment with both and see what works best for you. While music can help you switch off from the day, it can also serve as a distraction, meaning you get so caught up in the emotion of the music, you lose contact with what is real for you in the present moment.
- It's important that you're as comfortable as possible in Restorative yoga or your body won't fully relax, so spend as long as you need to position the props you're using in such a way that they don't restrict or create an imbalance in your body. Gather as many as you think you'll need, so you don't have to go looking around the house for another bolster or blanket once you begin, and remember to have a pair of warm socks and a blanket close by. We've used formal yoga props, but you can easily replace them with things you have around your home.
- Strap: a tie or scarf.
- Bolster: firm pillows or cushions.
- Blocks and bricks: hard-backed books.

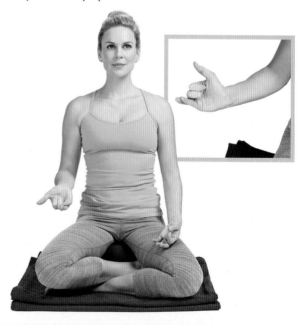

Pranayama

DOUBLE BREATHING

■ This calming yet energising breathing technique from Paramhansa Yogananda helps to oxygenate and detoxify your blood. Take a few breaths to establish a slow rhythm, then fully exhale through your mouth. Next, inhale strongly through your nose with a short, sharp intake of breath, then take a long, strong inhalation. The aim is to fill your lungs completely. Without pausing, exhale through both your nose and mouth, again with a short, then long exhalation. As you breathe out, make the sound: 'huh, huhhhhhh'. You're aiming to make the sound with your breath. Practise a few rounds, but don't do too much or you could hyperventilate. If you feel light-headed or agitated, stop and repeat another day, doing fewer rounds.

MOON BREATHING

■ Practise moon breathing when you want to feel calmer. Sitting comfortably, take a few breaths to centre yourself, then, with the back of your left hand resting on your left thigh, thumb and index finger touching, curl your right index and middle fingers into your right palm, and rest your right little finger on your right ring finger. Bring your right hand to your nose, place your thumb on the fleshy part of your right nostril and take your little and ring fingers to your left nostril. Inhale through your left nostril, then pause before closing it with your fingertips and releasing your thumb from your right nostril to exhale. Close your right nostril and release the left, breathing in through the left. Pause, close your left nostril and open your right, to exhale. Continue inhaling through the left and exhaling through the right for three minutes, release your hand, close your eyes and let your body feel the effects of the practice.

Meditation

MORNING MEDITATION

■ Replenish your system for a mindful day with this gentle exercise. Sitting comfortably with your eyes closed, take three deep breaths into your belly. Then let your attention float up to a point about an arm's-length above the crown of your head. Let your awareness rest there, then slowly begin to sense a growing white light in the surrounding area. If this doesn't come, you could visualise something white: a dove, a cloud, a snowy scene or a white object. Then, try to connect to the energy or feel of the colour, and hold it in your awareness as you also stay connected to the area above your head. Allow the feeling of light to be drawn down towards your body, feel it entering through the crown of your head and filling you up from head to toe, and sense it cascading in front and behind you, and to your sides. Be filled and surrounded by the feeling of white light. When ready to finish, bring your hands to prayer position in front of your heart, focus on the soles of your feet, noticing any sensations there, and open your eyes.

EVENING MEDITATION

■ This practice from Swami Sivananda will help you refresh your energy and let go of the day's cares. It uses the apana hand gesture, or mudra, which enables you to eliminate stale air from your lungs, promotes detoxification and also helps you release emotional 'toxins'. Lying on your back with your eyes closed and arms away from your sides, palms facing downwards, bring the tips of your middle and ring fingers together, then place the tip of your thumb where the two fingertips join. Let your index and little fingers be relaxed, but extended. Breathe softly and slowly through your nose, saying 'let' on the inhalation, 'go' on the exhalation. Respond to your words by sinking deeper into the mat on each exhalation.

Ado mukha svanasana

● Start on all-fours, knees beneath your hips, and place your hands a palm's-length in front of your shoulders, shoulder-width apart and fingers spread.
● Root through the base of your thumbs and index fingers, tuck under your toes and raise your knees off the mat, taking your tailbone back and up to lengthen your spine.
● Keeping your knees bent, root through your hands to extend your spine. Rotate

your upper arms externally and draw your shoulder blades down your spine. Lower your front ribs towards your thighs and release your neck.
● Gently draw one heel and then the other towards the mat, stretching out your hamstrings in a walking motion.
● Spread your toes and lower both heels towards the mat. Check your weight is evenly distributed through each foot and your inner arches lifted.

● Take five deep breaths then exhale and lower into Child's pose (p20).

VARIATION
Walk the dog
Help release your hamstrings by alternatively bending one knee and then the other as you extend the opposite heel towards the floor.

Good for:
• *Relieving extreme fatigue*
• *Aiding insomnia*
• *Calming your nervous system*
• *Reducing anxiety*

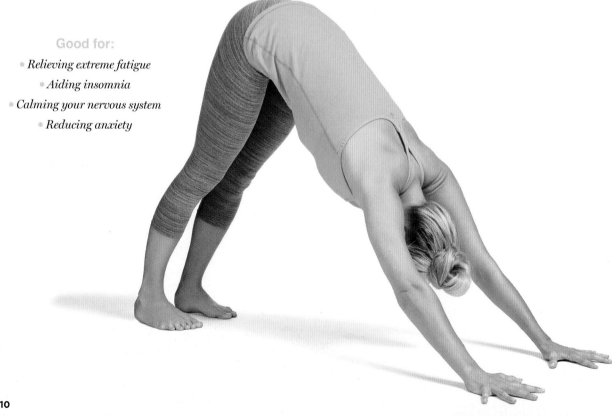

RESTORATIVE WIDE LEGGED STANDING FORWARD FOLD
Prasarita padottanasana

WHAT YOU NEED: BOLSTER OR PILLOWS, BLANKET

● Place a bolster lengthwise down the centre of your mat and rest a folded blanket on the end nearest to you. Stand in Mountain pose (p36) about 18 inches from the near end of the bolster, then step your feet wide with the inner edges parallel, toes spread and arches lifted. Anchor the outer edges of your feet into your mat.

● Rest your hands on your hips and, on an inhale, root through your feet to lengthen your spine. As you exhale, fold forwards from your hips and take your spine horizontal to the floor.

● Place your hands on the floor beneath your shoulders, then continue lengthening your spine as you inhale. Fold deeper as you exhale, allowing your forehead to slowly lower onto the folded blanket, walking your hands forwards as you do so.

● Draw up your kneecaps and engage your thighs, turning your inner thighs in slightly to open your sitting bones. Root your hands into the mat to draw your shoulders away from your ears.

● Breathe deeply and evenly for up to a minute, then walk your hands back under your shoulders and inhale to come back up.

Good for:

● *Resting your heart*
● *Calming your mind*
● *Soothing your sympathetic nervous system*
● *Stretching the back of your legs*

Tip

If you have tight hamstrings, bend your knees slightly. This pose will help to lengthen them naturally.

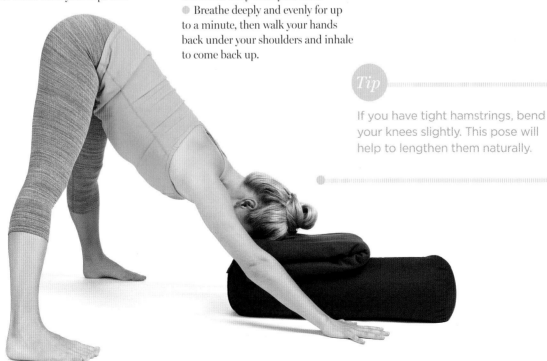

REVOLVED CHAIR
Parivrtta utkatasana

● Begin in Mountain pose (p36) with your feet up to hip-width apart, toes spread and arches lifted. On an inhale, ground through your feet as you sweep your arms up and forwards, palms facing, until your upper arms are level with your ears.

● Draw your navel to your spine and release your shoulder blades down your back. Lengthen through your fingertips, while drawing your arms back into your shoulder sockets. Keep your neck in line with your spine.

● As you exhale, bend your knees and lower your hips as if sitting down onto an imaginary chair. Simultaneously, take your hands to your heart, palms touching and twist to your right, resting your outside left elbow on your outside right knee.

● Continue rooting though your feet, draw your belly button to your spine and broaden your collar bones.

● Use the resistance of your elbow to lengthen your spine on the inhale, and deepen the twist on the exhale.

● Take five to 10 breaths, then inhale to come up to standing and exhale as you release your arms, before repeating on the other side.

Good for:

● *Relieving stiffness in your shoulders, spine and neck*

● *Opening your shoulders, chest and upper back*

● *Boosting your metabolism*

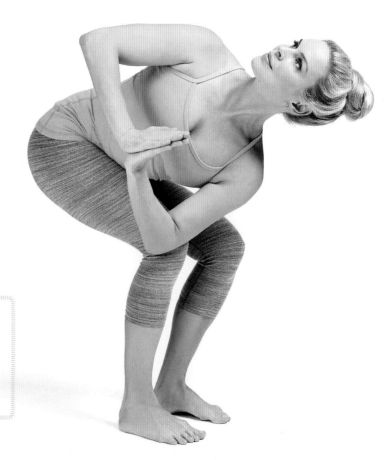

Tip

If one knee is in front of the other, draw your thigh bone back into your hip socket to keep your knees parallel.

BRIDGE
Setu bandha sarvangasana

WHAT YOU NEED: FOAM BRICK

Lie on your back, knees bent, feet on the floor hip-distance apart and parallel, directly beneath your knees. Rest your arms at your sides, palms facing down.

Inhale, ground through your feet and, on an exhale, tilt your tailbone up to gently peel your spine away from the floor, vertebra by vertebra.

Keep your thighs parallel, knees hip-distance apart and continue rooting through your feet to lift your chest. Roll your shoulders up, back and down, then lengthen the back of your neck.

Inhale and exhale, then take the foam brick and place it beneath your sacrum. Allow your weight to release into the brick while maintaining the lift in your chest.

Bring your hands together beneath you, interlink your fingers, index fingers pointed and snuggle your shoulders together. Focus on grounding through your feet to lift through your heart.

Take five deep breaths into your abdomen, then, on an exhale, slowly uncurl your spine to rest on the floor.

Good for:

- *Gently energising*
- *Calming your mind*
- *Resting your heart and nervous system*
- *Helping to reduce insomnia*

Tip

If keeping your thighs parallel places undue tension on your legs, loop a strap around your thighs, just above your knees.

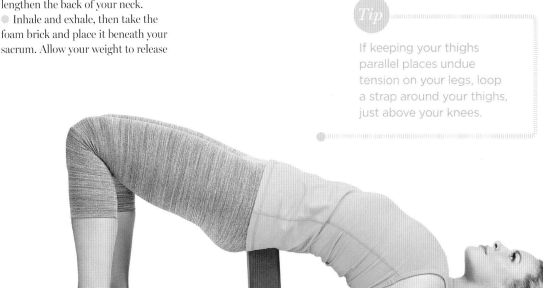

Supta baddha konasana

WHAT YOU NEED: TWO BLOCKS OR HARDBACK BOOKS

⬤ Place one block along the centreline of your mat, on its high end, and the other on its long side, as shown. Sit with your back to the lower block, and bring the soles of your feet together, letting your knees release out to the sides.

⬤ Place your hands either side of your hips and use them for support as you lower your back onto the bricks. If needed, adjust the bricks so the lower one is behind your heart, the higher one beneath your head.

⬤ Lift your chest, draw your shoulders back and down and take your hands to prayer position, resting your thumbs on your third eye. Alternatively, extend your arms overhead and rest your hands on the floor, palms together.

⬤ Take your attention to your breath, increasing the length of the exhale, and gently surrendering your weight to the supports beneath you.

⬤ Spend up to two minutes in the pose. Then, to come out, release your hands, rest your forearms on the floor beside you and press into the floor to gently bring yourself up to sitting.

Tip

If your legs feel strained, place a block or cushion beneath each knee.

Good for:

• *Grounding*
• *Opening your heart*
• *Quietening your mind*
• *Putting you in touch with your intuition*

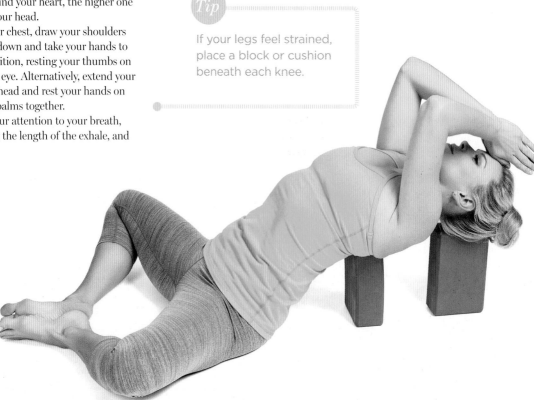

LEGS UP THE WALL
Viparita karani

WHAT YOU NEED: BOLSTER, BLANKET, EYE PILLOW

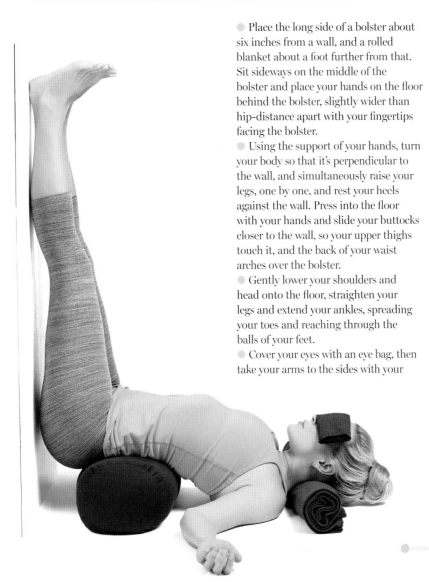

● Place the long side of a bolster about six inches from a wall, and a rolled blanket about a foot further from that. Sit sideways on the middle of the bolster and place your hands on the floor behind the bolster, slightly wider than hip-distance apart with your fingertips facing the bolster.

● Using the support of your hands, turn your body so that it's perpendicular to the wall, and simultaneously raise your legs, one by one, and rest your heels against the wall. Press into the floor with your hands and slide your buttocks closer to the wall, so your upper thighs touch it, and the back of your waist arches over the bolster.

● Gently lower your shoulders and head onto the floor, straighten your legs and extend your ankles, spreading your toes and reaching through the balls of your feet.

● Cover your eyes with an eye bag, then take your arms to the sides with your palms facing upwards. Breathe evenly for up to 10 minutes, feeling the expansion of your chest and abdomen on each inhale.

● To come out, bend your knees and place the soles of your feet against the wall. Raise your hips and push the bolster closer to the wall, then push away from the wall with your feet. Lower your hips to the floor and rest your legs on the bolster, then roll over to your right and gently come up to sitting.

Good for:

- *Easing tired legs*
- *Calming anxiety*
- *Regulating blood pressure*
- *Supporting slower breathing*

Tip

After coming out of the pose, spend a few moments in a comfortable seated position to allow your blood flow to return to normal.

WIDE-LEGGED SEATED FORWARD FOLD
Upavistha konasana

WHAT YOU NEED: BOLSTER, BLANKET

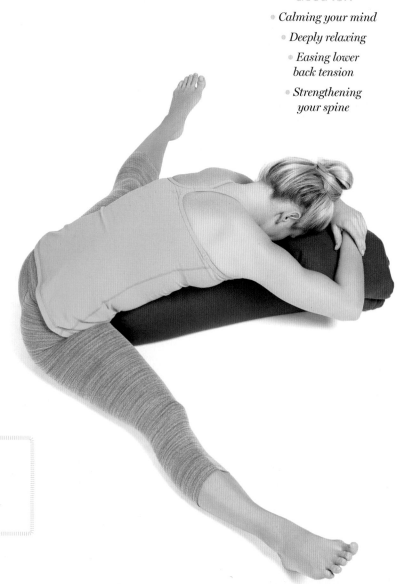

Good for:

- *Calming your mind*
- *Deeply relaxing*
- *Easing lower back tension*
- *Strengthening your spine*

● Sit on the floor. Take your legs wide, kneecaps facing the ceiling and feet resting on the centre of the back of each heel. Place a bolster in between your legs with a folded blanket at the far end.

● Use your hands to take the flesh of your buttocks backwards and away from your mid-line, so you can rest on the front of your sitting bones.

● Place your hands on the floor in front of you and, on an inhale, lengthen your front body by drawing your lower back forwards, then exhale and walk your hands forwards as you fold forwards from your hips, leading with your heart. If you feel a strain behind your knees, slightly bend your legs or place a folded towel under each knee.

● Fold your arms over the blanket and rest on your forehead for up to five minutes, breathing slowly and evenly.

● To come out, inhale as you walk your hands back to bring you up to sitting.

Tip

Aim to keep your kneecaps pointing towards the ceiling.

RESTORATIVE SUPINE TWIST

WHAT YOU NEED: BOLSTER

 Place a bolster lengthwise down the centre of your mat. Sit with your back to its short end, then snuggle your left buttock into the bolster, so your left thigh is parallel to it, your knees bent and the sole of your left foot resting against your right thigh.

 On an inhale, lengthen your spine and, as you exhale, twist to your left, walking your hands forwards as you fold from your hips to rest the centre of your chest over the bolster.

 Place your hands on top of each other on the bolster and rest your forehead on your hands, elbows on the floor. Draw your shoulder blades down your back to create space around your neck and let your neck be long.

 Breathe softly and evenly into your back and side ribs, releasing deeper into the twist on the exhale.

 After a couple of minutes, gently change sides. Then, when you're ready to come out of the pose, root through your hands to lift up, move the bolster to one side and rest in a comfortable seated position for a few breaths.

Good for:

- *Resting your brain*
- *Releasing muscles in your lower back*
- *Being mildly detoxifying*
- *Regulating your breathing*

Tip

To deepen the twist, turn your head in the opposite direction from your legs, and rest the side of your face on the bolster. You can place a folded blanket beneath your head/cheek if that feels more comfortable.

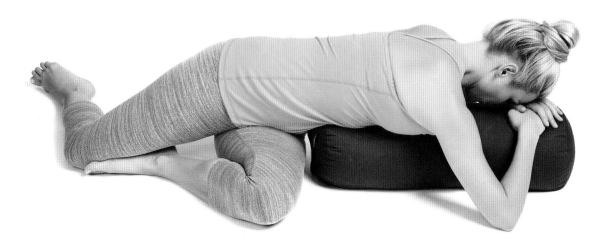

INVERTED STAFF POSE
Viparita dandasana

WHAT YOU NEED: BOLSTER, FOUR BLOCKS

Stagger the blocks on your mat, and rest a bolster against them with the short end resting on the floor next to the bottom block. Sit at the near end, with your buttocks close to the base of the bolster and your feet flat on the floor in front of you.

Gently and with control, and using the support of the floor beneath your feet, lie back on the bolster and walk your feet inwards so that it tilts back to balance on the blocks, as shown.

Extend your legs to balance on your heels, toes extended, and reach your hands overhead, arms straight and palms together, resting on the floor.

Remain in the pose for up to two minutes, breathing softly and evenly.

To come out, bend your knees and place your feet flat on the floor. Bring your hands to your hips, which will change your centre of gravity, and let the bolster rock forwards. Edge your buttocks forwards onto the floor to come up to sitting.

Good for:

- *Easing fatigue*
- *Releasing tight shoulders*
- *Opening your hip flexors*
- *Energising*

Tip

This is a strong pose. For a gentler variation, bend your knees and walk your feet in to bring your calves to a vertical position.

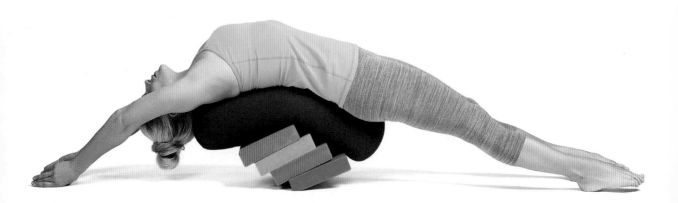

HEAD-TO-KNEE POSE
Janu sirsasana

WHAT YOU NEED: BOLSTER

Sit with your legs straight, feet together, ankles flexed and toes pointing to the ceiling. Fold your right leg in, so your right heel touches your pubic bone and your sole rests on your inner thigh. Draw your left hip back and your right knee forwards to square your hips.

Place a bolster lengthwise on top of your left leg, making sure your left ankle stays flexed. If this is uncomfortable for the knee of your extended leg, place a foam block beneath your knee. Spread your left toes and reach through the ball of your foot.

Place your hands either side of your left thigh, draw your navel to your spine, then inhale and root through your fingertips and sitting bones to lengthen your torso. As you exhale, lead with the crown of your head to fold forwards from your hips, taking your chest over the bolster.

Keeping your spine long and shoulder blades drawn in and down, fold your arms over the bolster and rest your forehead on your hands.

Breathe evenly and deeply for up to five minutes, then exhale to come up to sitting and repeat on the other side.

Good for:

- *Aiding insomnia*
- *Reducing anxiety*
- *Quietening your mind*
- *Easing back tension*

Tip

Fold forwards until you feel resistance, then take a few breaths in the pose. After a while your muscles will acclimatise to the stretch and you can fold deeper on an exhale.

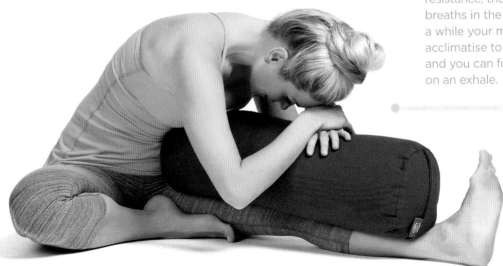

RESTORATIVE BUTTERFLY WITH BOLSTER
Supta baddha konasna

WHAT YOU NEED: BOLSTER, THREE BLANKETS, TWO FOAM BLOCKS, STRAP, EYE BAG

⬤ This is a super restorative version of Reclining bound angle pose, and it's worth setting up the props carefully to ensure you are completely comfortable. Place the bolster lengthwise on your mat.

⬤ Fold the blankets as shown and place one on the far end of the bolster and the other two at diagonal angles to it. Place the blocks either side.

⬤ Sit with your buttocks against the short edge of a bolster, and bring the soles of your feet together. Place the centre of an open strap around your lower back, bring the ends forwards and let them fall over your thighs and calves.

⬤ Take one end and loop it under the outside edges of both feet and fasten the strap so that the buckle doesn't push into your legs when you lie down. Rest each knee on a block.

⬤ Lower down onto the bolster, resting your head on the blanket. Place the eye bag over your eyes and rest your arms on the blankets, palms facing upwards.

⬤ Take time to get comfortable, adjusting your body as you need so you can relax fully. Take your attention to your breath, increasing the length of the exhale, and gently surrendering your weight to the supports beneath you.

⬤ Spend five to 10 minutes in the pose. Then, to come out, release the strap and use your hands to draw your knees together. Shift your bottom to the left, let your knees fall to your right and slowly roll your body over to the right. Take a few centring breaths, then use your hands to gently bring you up to sitting.

Good for:

⬤ *Gently stretching your legs*

⬤ *Calming your nervous system*

⬤ *Grounding yourself*

⬤ *Enhancing your breathing*

Tip
If your back feels uncomfortable, sit on a folded blanket to reduce the arch of your spine.

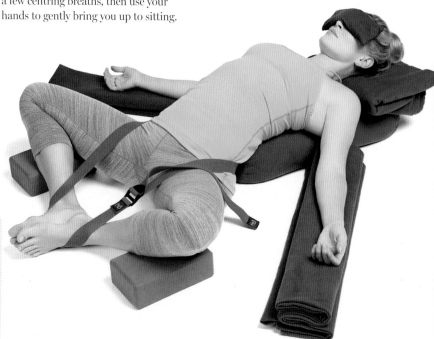

HEART-OPENING RELAXATION POSE
Savasana

WHAT YOU NEED: BOLSTER, BLANKET, EYE PILLOW

⦿ Place a bolster lengthwise along the centre of your mat, and fold a blanket over the far end. Have your eye bag close by.

⦿ Sit with your back to the bolster, with your buttocks about eight inches from the short end and extend your legs in front of you. Using your hands and then forearms to support you, gradually lower your back on to the bolster, so the end closest to you is level with your lower back ribs, as shown.

⦿ Rest your head back on the blanket, adjusting the height if you need to by placing a block underneath the blanket. Let your arms fall out to the sides, palms facing upwards. Make any minor adjustments you need so there is no strain on your body.

⦿ Gently connect to your breath and surrender your weight to the earth. Rest here for as long as is comfortable, up to 20 minutes.

⦿ To come out of the pose, slowly wriggle your fingers and toes, remove your eye bag and bend your knees, bringing your feet to the floor near your buttocks. Gently roll over to your right side and rest in a foetal position for a moment or two before using your hands to help you come up to sitting.

Good for:

Opening your upper chest

Aiding your breathing

Resting your legs

Calming your mind

Tip

To deepen the relaxation visualise you're standing on a beach with your feet in the sea, covering your ankles. Watch each wave gently flow around your feet, then draw backwards into the vast sea, matching the movement of the waves with your breath.

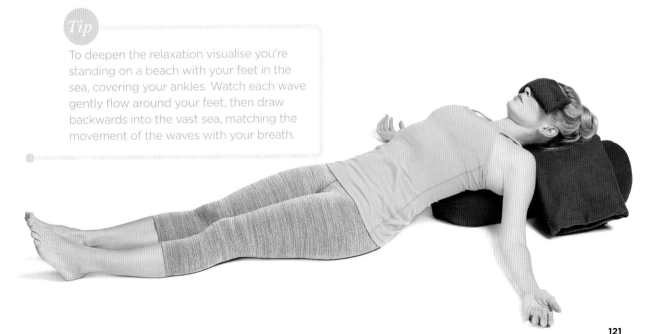

THE RESTORATIVE
AM sequence

Wake up
your body

This sequence is designed to get your body moving slowly and gently first thing in the morning and to help replenish your energy if you've had a poor night's sleep. Unless otherwise stated, aim to spend about five to 10 breaths in each pose, but listen to your instincts, staying longer if it feels right for your body, coming out of the pose sooner if you feel you have spent enough time there.

Breathe softly and gently into your abdomen for each posture.

1 Downward dog (p110)

2 Wide-legged standing forward fold (p111)
Up to one minute

3 Revolved chair (p112)

4 Bridge with block (p113)

5 Restorative butterfly with blocks (p114)
Up to two minutes

6 Heart-opening relaxation (p121)
Five to seven minutes

The moves

START

Warm-up
Extended child's pose (p55), with side stretch

Cat/Cow (p20), into free form Reclining twist (p21)

Pranayama
Single nostril breathing (p109)

Sun salute
Moon salute I (p28)

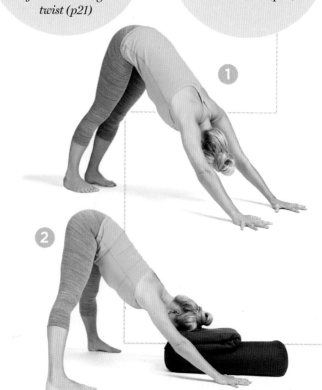

① ②

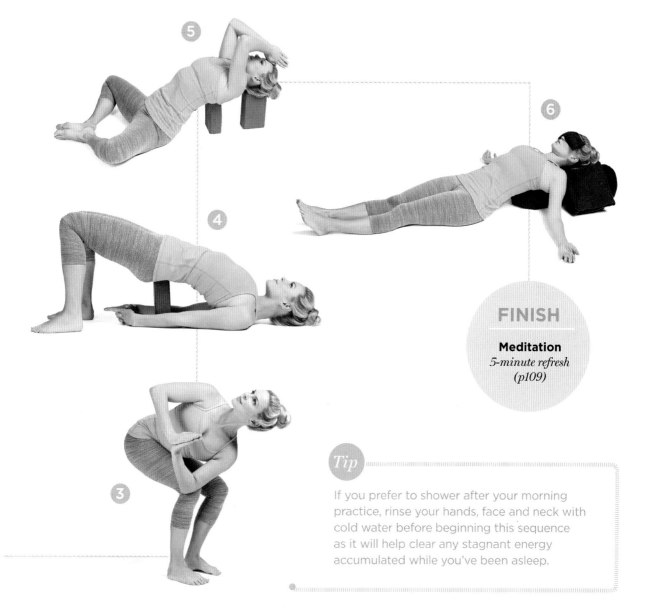

FINISH

Meditation
5-minute refresh
(p109)

Tip

If you prefer to shower after your morning practice, rinse your hands, face and neck with cold water before beginning this sequence as it will help clear any stagnant energy accumulated while you've been asleep.

THE RESTORATIVE
PM sequence

Wind down
and relax

This soothing evening practice will help prepare your body for sleep by releasing physical tension in your shoulders, spine, hips and hamstrings, while also calming your mind and relaxing your nervous system. Breathe softly and gently into your abdomen for each posture, making the exhale longer than the inhale to increase the relaxation response even further. Make yourself as comfortable as possible – you may prefer to practise on a cosy rug instead of a yoga mat – and have a blanket close by in case you need it. Use the times suggested as a guideline, adjusting them according to your needs on the day.

1 Wide-legged forward fold (p116)

2 Restorative twist (p117)
Up to two minutes each side

3 Inverted staff (p118)
Up to two minutes

4 Head-to-knee (p119)
Up to five minutes each side

5 Restorative butterfly with bolster (p120)
Five to 10 minutes

6 Heart-opening relaxation (p121)
Ten to 15 minutes

The moves

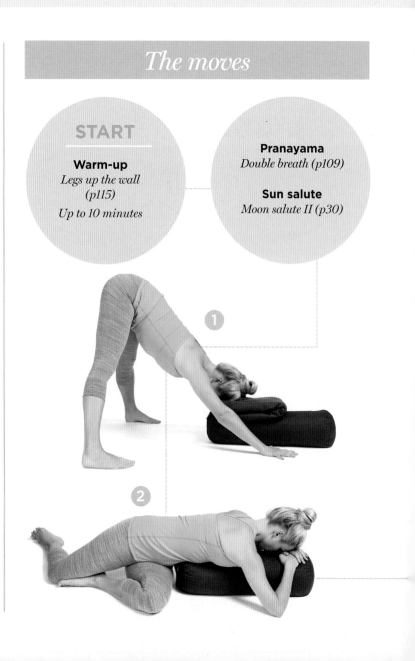

START

Warm-up
Legs up the wall (p115)
Up to 10 minutes

Pranayama
Double breath (p109)

Sun salute
Moon salute II (p30)

① ②

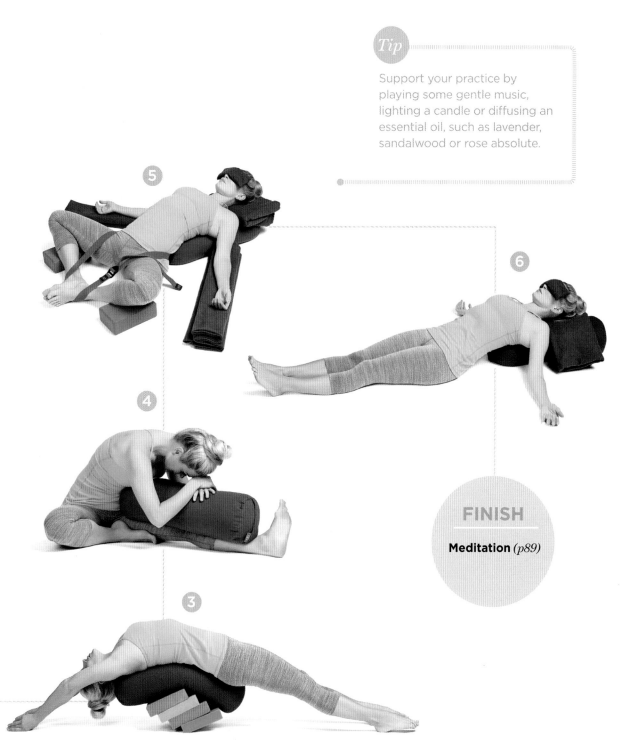

Tip

Support your practice by playing some gentle music, lighting a candle or diffusing an essential oil, such as lavender, sandalwood or rose absolute.

FINISH

Meditation *(p89)*

DIRECTORY

Apparel

ACTIVE IN STYLE
activeinstyle.com

ASQUITH
asquithlondon.com

EVERY SECOND COUNTS
everysecondcounts.co.uk

FROMYOGA
fromclothing.com

ILU
ilufitwear.com

LULULEMON
lululemon.co.uk

MADEBYYOGIS
yogaclicks.store

MANDUKA
manduka.com

M LIFE
mlifelondon.com

NOBALLS
noballs.co.uk

PURE LIME
purelimeshop.com

STYLE PB
stylepb.com

SWEATY BETTY
sweatybetty.com

**UNDER THE
SAME SUN**
underthesamesun.se

WELLICIOUS
wellicious.com

Equipment

EKOTEX YOGA
ekotexyoga.co.uk

GAIAM
gaiameurope.se

HOLISTIC SILK
holisticsilk.com

MADEBYYOGIS
yogaclicks.store

MANDUKA
manduka.com

YOGA BLISS
yogabliss.co.uk

YOGA MATTERS
yogamatters.com

YOGA STUDIO
yogastudio.co.uk

Find a teacher

**THE BRITISH
WHEEL OF YOGA**
bwy.org.uk

YOGA ALLIANCE
yogaalliance.co.uk

JUDITH HANSON LASATER
judithhansonlasater.com

SARAH POWERS
sarahpowers.com

SHIVA REA
shivarea.com

TRIYOGA
triyoga.co.uk

YOGA WITH SIMON LOW
simonlow.com

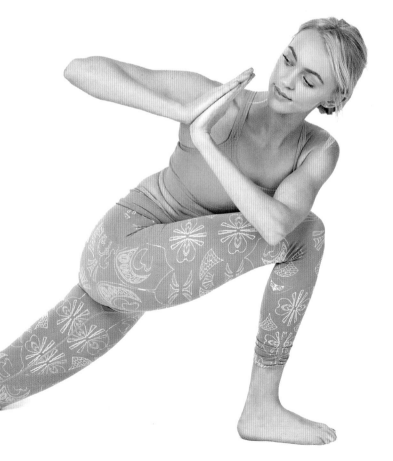

DIRECTORY

Online yoga classes

EKART YOGA
ekhartyoga.com

MOVEMENT FOR MODERN LIFE
movementformodernlife.com

GAIA
gaia.com

YOGAGLO
yogaglo.com

YOGAIA
yogaia.com

Organisations

IYENGAR YOGA
iyi.org.uk

RESTORATIVE YOGA
Judithhansonlasater.com

SIVANANDA YOGA
sivananda.org

VINYASA YOGA
shivarea.com

YIN YOGA
yinyoga.com

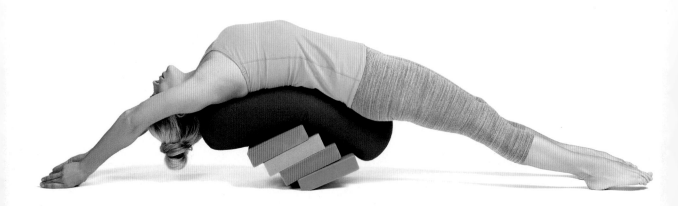

FAREWELL.

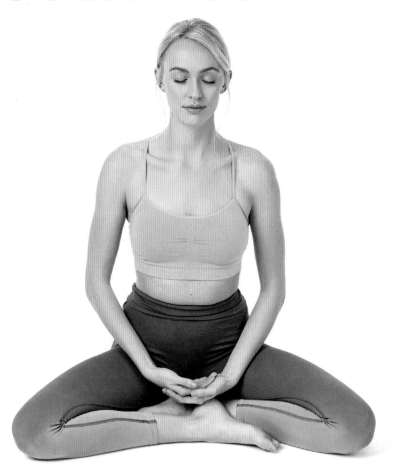

We hope you've enjoyed working your way through *Everyday Yoga*, and are reaping the benefits of a regular yoga practice. Now that you have more understanding of the yoga styles in this book, you can tune in to your deeper needs on the day of your practice and choose to work with the style that best suits you. Whether it's increasing flexibility with Yin yoga, combatting work stress with Restorative or building strength with Vinyasa, you can turn to the relevant pages and find the guidance you need. But don't stop there, why not sign up for a six-week Iyengar class or drop in to a Restorative session at your local studio and chill with others? The more you allow the benefits of yoga to support and transform your mind and body, the richer your life will be.

Eve